PREGNANCY

DIET

and

CANCER

A HIGH FAT DIET DURING PREGNANCY MAY PROGRAM YOUR UNBORN CHILD FOR CANCER LATER IN LIFE

by

Bruce E. Walker, M.D., Ph.D

McCUAIG PUBLISHING COMPANY

Published by
McCuaig Publishing Company
Box 235
Bath, Michigan, 48808

Notice: The purpose of this book is to increase
public awareness of the issues addressed so as to
encourage public debate and government action.
A further purpose is to increase patient
understanding of health issues and thus facilitate
communication between patients and their
physicians. It is not intended to be used as the
basis for self-prescription and treatment. Neither
the publishing company nor the author of this
book can take responsibility for adverse health
outcomes arising from self-treatment.

Library of Congress Catalog Card Number:
89-91643

ISBN 0-9622878-0-6

CONTENTS

Acknowledgements

I wish to sincerely thank the many people who have helped me in a variety of ways during the development of this book. Among my professional colleagues, I am especially pleased to recognize the help of two outstanding physicians. Dr. Bruce H. Drukker has drawn upon his extensive clinical knowledge of normal and abnormal functioning of the female reproductive system to offer me valuable suggestions. The insights of Dr. Albert W. Sparrow have been important to me since they were based on extensive experience with theories and applications in the area of diet and health. Much of the help I have received has come from people who have offered me the perspective of the average reader. Some members of the Grand Rapids chapter of DES Action have worked hard to develop this perspective and I am pleased to specifically thank Pamela VanderBee, Gloria Janes, Ande Jones, Anne O'Neill and Debra Wilkerson. Others who have contributed in various ways are Lori Kurth, Dianne Fullerton and Sally Walker. Finally, I wish to thank someone who has shared this enterprise with me from beginning to end - my wife, Lois.

Chapter One

CANCER FROM DIETARY FAT EARLY IN LIFE

Current research supports the conclusion that a high fat diet during pregnancy programs the unborn baby for cancer later in life. Direct evidence for this relationship has come from an experiment in which pregnant mice were given diets that were low in fat, or high in fat. Then the pups were raised to adults and the numbers of diet-related tumors were counted. The mice whose mothers were on a low fat diet had very few diet-related tumors. The mice whose mothers were on a high fat diet had a lot of these tumors. Faced with this evidence, should any woman ever again go through pregnancy on a high fat diet? Yet, an excessively low fat diet might be harmful, because there are essential fatty acids in fat. Also fat is used in the development of the brain and many other tissues. Why not develop a fat-controlled diet to stay within a safe range of dietary fat consumption? Since it takes time to develop a fat-controlled diet, and since the critical period for cancer is early in pregnancy, the diet should be started well before the onset of pregnancy. Unfortunately, the onset of pregnancy is often not predictable. The problem would be solved if every woman of childbearing age went on a fat-controlled diet.

Excuses

Learning about a fat-controlled diet and then developing one for your own use takes time and effort. Most of us are already swamped with current demands and are quite resistant to adding another major project. It would be very attractive if someone could provide you with an excuse for ignoring this new problem. Skeptics and critical experts will rise to the occasion. "Wasn't the final link in the high fat story based on only a single experiment with animals? It must be confirmed by other laboratories before we can take it seriously." "No one has directly proven that a low fat diet during human pregnancy will stop cancer in the offspring." "Let's wait a few years to see how this story stands up."

The Hour of Truth

Delaying pregnancies is not a practical option. There were almost four million babies born in the U.S. last year and there will not be any fewer this year. If the evidence grows steadily stronger with the years that a high fat diet programs the unborn baby for cancer, your child will eventually ask: "Mom, did you go on a fat-controlled diet when you were having me?" How would your excuses sound then? It would be better to thoroughly explore the evidence now than to have missed this opportunity to give your child a major head start in avoiding cancer.

The Purpose of this Book

I expect the public media will have reported my research by the time this book is released. Surely many people will have read or heard a brief report and wish to learn more about the issue. A major purpose of this book is to provide a resource for reviewing the issue and deciding whether to take action. The information presented here should be used in conjunction with all other available sources to reach a well informed decision consistent with the level of knowledge that exists at the time the decision is being made. The second purpose of the book is to provide information on diet management to help those who decide to control intake of fat in preparation for pregnancy. The decision should be reached in consultation with your physician.

Dr. Koop's Recommendation.

The Surgeon General's Report on Nutrition and Health, prepared by a distinguished committee of scientists, was released during the summer of 1988. In his introduction to this report, Dr. Koop highlighted their most important conclusion, namely, that overconsumption of certain dietary components is now a major concern for Americans.

The greatest danger comes from a disproportionate consumption of foods high in fat. Therefore, the main recommendation in this government report is to reduce the amount of fat in the diet. Consuming less fat should reduce the risk of coronary heart disease, diabetes, obesity, and some types of cancer. Since my book provides a thorough explanation of how to reduce consumption of dietary fat in Chapter Three through Chapter Six, it can be used as a means of understanding how to achieve the most important goal set by Dr. Koop. Although the major focus of my book is cancer, Chapter Eight on weight control and Chapter Nine on family meals provide further information on other diseases and nutritional factors discussed in the Surgeon General's report.

How Much Fat is Too Much?

The average dietary intake of fat in this country is 37% of calories from fat. Therefore, if the average American woman decides to continue on her current diet during pregnancy, she has decided to expose her unborn child to this high level of fat and to accept whatever damage this might cause. Yet, previous warnings on dangers of eating too much fat have typically been directed to middle-aged men at risk for heart attack. At what other stages of life should human beings be protected from high fat?

Who Should Avoid A High Fat Diet

The Surgeon General's report does have a section on Maternal and Child Nutrition. Some statements are of a general nature, such as "well nourished mothers produce healthier children" and that there should be "intake of sufficient energy and nutrients to attain optimal nutritional status, including appropriate weight before pregnancy and adequate weight gain during pregnancy" to assure a healthy child. Limits set for inadequate and excessive prepregnancy weight were "below 85% or above 120% of standard weight for height." Concerning fat specifically, adolescents were advised to eat sufficient quantities of low-fat, nutritious foods. Advice offered for earlier stages of life was that "Parents should guide their children in developing positive eating behaviors and on age-appropriate food patterns that meet nutritional requirements but avoid excessive intake of fat, sodium, and sugar" and that "breast milk is the optimal food for infants." No comment was made on level of fat intake for pregnant women.

What About Diet Before Birth?

Is it believable that dietary fat is very important from childhood through old age, but doesn't matter before birth? The period of human development from the fertilized egg to the newborn baby is one of tremendous change. The conceptus goes from a single cell to billions of cells. All the major tissues and organs of the body come into existence during this time. Why was this dynamic period of life passed over by the committee in making its recommendations concerning dietary fat? Presumably, because of the paucity of information concerning dietary fat and pregnancy in the scientific literature. They did admit to "gaps in our knowledge of nutrition" and suggested future research on "The effects of maternal nutrition on the health of the developing fetus."

Should Any Recommendation Be Made for Pregnant Women?

Undoubtedly, the scientists and physicians who prepared the Surgeon General's report were well aware of the sensitivity of the unborn baby to being upset by a wide variety of factors. Yet, they had no direct evidence on which to base a recommendation. My research on dietary fat during pregnancy was incomplete when Dr. Koop's report was issued and so could not have influenced that report. Is one experiment on mice enough to justify a new recommendation? Should the work be confirmed by other laboratories and studied from many different perspectives before being released to the public? The problem is that silence is a recommendation. Failure to challenge the high fat diet consumed by most pregnant women in this country is not any different in outcome than specifically recommending a high fat diet. In fact, the diet often recommended by professionals on the basis of being "nutritious" can be even higher in fat than the average 37% fat diet.

The Issue Must Be Faced!

Silence on this issue is no longer justified. It has taken me five years to complete one experiment with mice on dietary fat during pregnancy. Waiting another five to ten years for more experiments of this nature means accepting that another twenty to forty million babies will be born without protection from exposure to high fat. I believe the public has a right to know now that dietary fat during pregnancy is an issue. Furthermore, the public should have convenient access to information that supports a recommendation for lowering fat intake during pregnancy. Similarly, justification (if any) for the typical high fat American diet during pregnancy should be clearly explained and documented.

What Evidence Supports High Fat?

I am not aware of any scientific evidence to support a recommendation for high dietary fat intake during pregnancy. Therefore, this book does not present both sides of the issue. All the data I will present are in favor of reducing fat intake. If anyone knows of good scientific information already available to support a diet of 37% fat, or higher, they should speak out.

How To Use This Book

The remainder of this chapter discusses the evidence from human studies supporting the idea that some cancers are caused by exposure to dietary fat early in life, probably during pregnancy. The second chapter discusses the evidence from animal experiments that a high fat diet during pregnancy programs the offspring for cancer later in life. The rest of this chapter is somewhat technical. Chapter Two is quite technical. In contrast, the chapters on diet control should be reasonably easy to follow, so don't get discouraged too soon. A good compromise would be to read the technical material without becoming too concerned about thoroughly understanding some of the details. If the theoretical issues become too confusing, watch for trends of scientific opinion in the public media and keep in touch with your physician.

The Causes of Cancer

Some people say so many things cause cancer it's impossible to avoid them all, so why bother with any! If we include all the chemicals that have been injected into rodents and found to cause cancer, then the list would be very long. As far as the substances that have actually been proven to cause cancer in people, the list is surprisingly short. Tobacco heads the list as a potent human carcinogen - potent in terms of the number of people who develop cancer from it. Alcohol, especially when combined with tobacco, is believed to be a significant cancer producer. Certain chemicals involving mainly industrial exposure, like asbestos and aniline dyes, produced many cancers in the past. Natural estrogens used to relieve postmenopausal symptoms and synthetic estrogens like DES have been linked to genital tract cancers in women. Ultraviolet rays in sunlight cause skin cancer.

The real issue for most of us is this: What agents or habits are most likely to cause fatal cancer in the average person? Authoritative estimates have been published and they agree on the general categories. Tobacco is commonly listed as accounting for 30% of all human cancers. Surprisingly, less than 1% of fatal cancers are attributed to industrial products and just 2% to pollution. The only other large category besides tobacco is diet. One estimate attributed 40% of cancers in men and 60% of cancers in women to diet. You might assume the culprit in diet to be some chemical contaminating our food supply. When a committee of the National Academy of Sciences reviewed scientific publications on diet and cancer they arrived at a very different conclusion. They decided that the evidence was strongest for fat as the major cause of cancer in the diet.

International Differences in Cancer

Dramatic differences in cancer rates between

certain countries have been established. We might
be tempted to blame this on genetic differences in
susceptibility to cancer between groups of people.
Yet when people migrate to a new country they
tend to develop the cancer rate of that country.
Something in their new environment is
responsible for the cancer. Of all the changes
that occur with migration, the change of diet
seems to be the most likely explanation for the
change in cancer rate. When breast cancer
frequency is compared to dietary fat intake for a
variety of countries, there is a constant relation.
As the amount of fat in the typical diet increases
from country to country, the rate of breast cancer
increases proportionately. A similar correlation
exists for colon cancer, prostate cancer, ovarian
cancer and endometrial cancer of the uterus.
Almost 500,000 new cases of these 5 cancers are
expected in 1988. If eating less fat would
significantly reduce their incidence, this would be
a tremendous accomplishment. Such a hope has
caused the National Cancer Institute to urge all
Americans to cut back on the amount of fat they
eat.

Contradictions

Unfortunately, there are contradictions in the
fat and cancer story. When the diets within a
country have been analyzed for fat content and
these results compared with frequency of breast
cancer, the strong correlation seen with
international comparisons has not shown up. For

example, the nuns at certain monasteries in England eat a low fat diet. When their rate of breast cancer was compared with that of nulliparous (never-pregnant) women in the general population on the usual high fat diet, there was no difference. The scientists who reported this study pointed out that the nuns entered the convent only after they had reached adult age. If the critical period for high fat exposure is early in life, then the nuns would be expected to have as high a cancer rate as the rest of the population.

Despite these discouraging results, the possibility of reducing breast cancer frequency by dietary change is so attractive that the National Cancer Institute planned a massive experiment costing over one hundred million dollars. They would persuade a large group of women to live on a low fat diet, then follow them to record their breast cancer rate compared to a group on the usual high fat diet. Meanwhile, the results of another large study have been announced. About 90,000 U.S. nurses were tracked for 4 years to compare their consumption of fat with diagnosis of breast cancer. No correlation was found between amount of fat eaten and number of breast cancer cases diagnosed. Again the authors pointed out that this study did not exclude a possible effect of dietary fat before adulthood.

One exception to the failure to find a correlation between diet and cancer within a country was a study performed in Hawaii. The researchers compared diet and cancer between the five main ethnic groups in Hawaii, namely, native Hawaiians, Caucasians, Japanese, Chinese, and Filipinos. They found that breast, uterine and prostate cancer correlated with fat intake. This finding is not necessarily in contradiction to the other studies just mentioned. In the study of nurses, the differences in diet were probably due to adult preferences and did not necessarily reflect what foods the nurses were exposed to before they were adults. In contrast, the Hawaiian study reflected dietary differences between ethnic groups that were probably stable throughout the lives of the individuals. So these results were consistent with a dietary fat effect early in life.

Other Risk Factors

The characteristics of women who get breast cancer have been compared with those who are free of the disease. Consistent differences relate to the functional history of the reproductive system. A higher risk of cancer is associated with decreased fertility, late menopause and early menarche (menarche is the first menstrual period of a young girl). Since one of these risk factors is already established by puberty, critical events must be happening early in life to program for breast cancer later in life. Similar risk factors have been established for uterine and ovarian cancers. These risk factors probably involve the balance of hormones in the woman's body, especially estrogen. So conditions which determine the balance of hormones in the body apparently are established early in life. Another risk factor involves body size. According to one group of investigators, this association of stature and frame size with risk of breast cancer suggests a potential role for early nutrition in the development of cancer.

How Early is Earlier?

As you can see, the evidence keeps pointing to events taking place earlier than the adult stage of life. Studies on human populations have not given much hint about which part of preadult life constitutes the critical period. Is it the teenage years, childhood, or prenatal (prenatal means before birth)? Some useful information comes from comparison of cancer rates between immigrant Japanese women and their American-born daughters. Immigrating from Japan to the U.S.A. means moving from an environment where reproductive system cancer (breast, uterine, and ovarian cancer) is low to an area in which the average breast cancer rate is more than five times as high, ovarian cancer is four times as high and uterine cancer (excluding cervical) is ten to twenty times as high. Currently, Japanese women living in this country have an intermediate cancer rate. However, when the rates for immigrant and American-born Japanese women are separated, much of the increase comes from the Japanese women who were born here. Is this because the immigrant

Japanese women were on a high fat American diet by the time they became pregnant in this country?

The obvious answer is to inquire about diet and other events during pregnancy and compare this information with the cancer rates in the offspring. The problem with looking for this information is that cancer tends to occur late in life. Trying to find out what a person's mother ate 40 to 60 years ago when she was pregnant is very difficult. One group of scientists took advantage of the fact that testicular cancer appears relatively early, reaching maximum frequency between the ages of 20 and 40. To reduce the time gap even more, they studied only men under age 30 with testicular cancer. Then they were able to question the men's mothers concerning events during pregnancy, especially whether they were given any hormone drugs. As suspected, the mothers whose sons had developed testicular cancer were more likely to have been given estrogenic hormones during pregnancy. Also, they tended to weigh more than the average woman. Increased fat tissue is known to increase the amount of estrogen in the body, so hormones seem to have been the common factor.

The DES Story

The risk factors for testicular cancer hint that the period of prenatal development may be the early stage of life when cancer gets programmed. However, a much stronger story has arisen from studies of another type of cancer seen early in life. Almost 20 years ago Boston physicians noticed a cluster of rare cancers in 8 young women. They all had a glandular type of cancer in the lower genital tract. Since the patients were only 14 to 22 years of age, the physicians were able to follow their medical histories all the way back to birth and to question their mothers about drugs taken during pregnancy. All the mothers had received a synthetic estrogen medicine called diethylstilbestrol, or DES. This correlation has been confirmed many times since then. A total of about a million women have been exposed to DES prenatally. The term "DES daughters" is used to identify this large group of women.

In addition to causing cancer, the DES has changed the hormone balance in many DES daughters. They also are at increased risk of pregnancy failure. Tracking back to the time their mothers took the drug revealed that the critical period for prenatal exposure to DES was during the third to fourth months of pregnancy, and perhaps even as early as the end of the second month. So now we have evidence that the critical period for disrupting development of the reproductive system and programming offspring for cancer later in life is during the early part of pregnancy. There is no evidence that such an effect can be derived from exposures during childhood, or during the teenage period.

Now there is enough information to tie the whole story together. Using breast cancer as an example, risk for breast cancer is already recognizable by menarche, so at least some of the events that establish this risk must have already occurred by then. The logical time for them to happen is early pregnancy, as shown by the DES effect. Exposure to a high fat diet sometime early in life increases the risk of breast cancer. The time to expect this effect is when the risk factors are being established. Therefore, the most critical time for high fat diet to increase cancer risk should be during early pregnancy. Notice that this conclusion can be reached without any reference to animal experimentation. The conclusion is reached by reasoning rather than direct proof. Nevertheless, it is sufficiently convincing to justify considering a determined avoidance of high fat diets during pregnancy without necessarily waiting for further evidence. Since the critical period is during early pregnancy, all women of childbearing age should consider starting to develop a fat-controlled diet now.

Chapter Two

HIGH DIETARY FAT CAUSES CANCER IN THE OFFSPRING

Studying laboratory rodents has some important advantages. Their environment can be closely controlled so that the only difference between two experimental groups is the factor we are studying. Mice go through their complete life cycle from conception to the illnesses of old age in just 2 to 3 years. Their old age illnesses, especially cancer, are similar to those of people. The disadvantage of using mice and rats is that they are also different in many ways from people. It is very important to find out how similar, or different they are in regard to the disease being studied.

Animal experimentation is especially useful in finding explanations for biologic phenomena that are not understood on the basis of human studies. For example, in the previous chapter we saw a great opportunity to prevent cancer by lowering dietary fat, according to studies comparing countries with different eating habits. Yet, differences in amount of fat eaten by adults within a country did not clearly affect reproductive cancer rates. Thus, the sensitive period must be early in life. Studies on human exposure to DES indicated that the early prenatal stage of development (third and fourth months of pregnancy) was the critical period in respect to programming offspring for cancer. Therefore, this is a likely time for diet to be having its effect also. Yet, we do not have much evidence that this is the only sensitive time. Secondly, we do not understand what happens at that time to cause cancer later. Thirdly, we do not have direct evidence that changing the amount of fat in the diet during early pregnancy will change cancer frequency later in life. Fortunately these issues have already been resolved to a surprising degree by animal experimentation.

The Fetal Period

Prenatal development of the baby is described using two terms. During the first two months of human pregnancy the baby is referred to as an embryo. From the third month to birth, the baby is called a fetus. Actually, the term baby does not apply until the time of birth. Some understanding of cancer programming early in life was gained as long ago as the 1940's. Injection of a cancer-causing chemical through the uterus into the fluid surrounding mouse fetuses caused them to develop cancer, but not until they reached the adult stage of life. In another experiment, a chemical was injected into the mother and it programmed the fetus for cancer later in life. These types of experiments have been performed many times since. It is now well established that the most sensitive period for prenatal cancer programming is the fetal stage and the usual time for the cancer to appear is well into the adult stage of life. Typically, these same chemicals will cause cancer at other stages of the life cycle too, but the sensitivity can be very different. For example, a single tiny dose of DES given during the fetal period will program mice for a high frequency of uterine cancer when they grow old. To accomplish the same effect by treatment during the juvenile, or adult stage of life requires large doses given repeatedly over a long time.

Risk Factors

Experiments performed around 1940 also gave some hint about risk factors. When rat fetuses were exposed to large doses of estrogens, including DES, the development of their reproductive system was abnormal. One outcome was that when the rats grew up they had structural changes in their ovaries that indicated they had a disturbed hormonal balance with an excess of estrogen. Clinical studies during the same decade were leading physicians to believe that a significant cause of reproductive system cancer in women was a disturbed hormone balance involving a similar structural change in the ovary and an excess of estrogen.

Genital Tract Cancer

A direct link between reproductive system

development and cancer was established in 1963. DES was injected into newborn mice and they developed genital tract cancer when they grew up. This may seem to contradict the evidence that the fetal period is the most sensitive period. Actually, this is not a contradiction, because the mouse is born at a much earlier stage of development than the human baby. In the mouse, the reproductive tract is still developing at birth and the newborn mouse is equivalent to about the third to fourth month of human pregnancy. The authors of this study recommended that physicians look for the cause of human genital tract cancer among the events occurring early in life.

The DES Animal Model

The publication in 1971 of evidence that exposing human fetuses to DES was causing cancer in female offspring has had both practical and theoretical consequences of great importance. This was the first example of something happening to the pregnant woman which led to cancer in the offspring after they grew up. Human studies established that prenatal exposure to DES caused a high frequency of genital tract abnormalities called vaginal adenosis, transverse vaginal ridges and cervical metaplasia. The DES exposure also increased susceptibility to the common type of cervical cancer as well as producing the DES type of glandular cancer. As mentioned before, DES caused pregnancy failures in DES daughters. All of these changes have been duplicated in a mouse model. This establishes that the mouse model is relevant to the human DES problem. The model is also appropriate for studying the general issue of maternal-fetal interactions leading to cancer. New discoveries with this model need to be taken very seriously, even though the possibility will always exist that people may react differently.

DES and Diet

Does the DES story have any relevance to the problem of dietary fat and cancer? As already mentioned, it has helped in establishing at least one sensitive period for programming reproductive system cancer. Secondly, it has provided a model to study the mechanism by which certain cancers are programmed to appear later in life. The issue of how DES causes cancer has not been settled. Yet, some valuable leads have appeared that will be useful in considering a possible dietary effect. One discovery is that the mouse model develops a high frequency of pituitary gland tumors late in life. These tumors contain many cells that secrete a hormone called prolactin. This observation ties the prenatal induction of cancer into a lot of other very important work.

Pituitary Tumors

The pituitary gland is situated at the base of the brain. It secretes hormones that control the function of other hormone-producing glands like the ovary. Tumors of glands like the pituitary can arise from overworking the gland. If the pituitary is being overworked we can expect hormones to be out of balance. Abnormal hormone exposures, like excess estrogen, are believed to be a major cause of human reproductive system cancer. Therefore, DES may be causing cancer indirectly by upsetting the function of the pituitary gland. Malfunction of the pituitary gland then creates the abnormal hormone levels that produce cancer. This leaves one more question. What controls the working of the pituitary gland? The secretion of the pituitary gland is controlled by a part of the brain called the hypothalamus. The hypothalamus is at the base of the brain right above the pituitary gland and constantly sends messages down to it through special pathways. Of course, this just pushes the questioning one step further. How could DES, and maybe diet, influence the working of the hypothalamus? Fortunately, a lot is known about this matter.

The Hypothalamus

Over the past several decades many experiments on the development of the hypothalamus have been performed in rodents. Remember that the time of development we are interested in for rodents is late pregnancy and the newborn period. This is the same period that the hypothalamus is going through a critical phase of development. If hormone balance is upset at that time (for example, by giving DES) then the hypothalamus develops abnormally. If the hypothalamus of a baby female rat is exposed to an excess estrogen effect at this time, the rat will go through puberty normally. Then its hormone balance will become upset and it will eventually develop an ovary with structural changes reflecting further irregularities in hormone balance.

Do any of these effects occur in the human population? Although DES daughters are still too young to expect many pituitary tumors, there are anecdotical reports about an increased incidence of these tumors and elevated levels of the prolactin hormone. Fortunately, pituitary tumors tend not to be dangerous. The issue is important mainly for understanding the action of DES. Thus, both animal and clinical studies support the hypothesis that DES programs for cancer later in life by upsetting the differentiation of the hypothalamus, which in turn leads to hormone changes and cancer.

Designing a Diet Experiment

In 1984 I decided it would be worth testing the effects of a high fat diet during pregnancy on mice. The first issue was to decide what would make a sensitive model for testing a dietary effect. The cancer which seemed most affected by international differences in dietary fat was endometrial cancer of the uterus (endometrium is the inner lining of the uterus). The rate for this cancer in the U.S. is 10 to 20 times higher than in Japan. Yet rodents almost never get this type of cancer. If they are very resistant to it, then a subtle agent like dietary fat might be too weak to break down the natural resistance of the rodent to uterine endometrial cancer. On the other hand, fetal mice exposed prenatally to DES develop a high incidence of endometrial cancer late in life. The problem with this model is that a dose of the potent DES hormone would be injected at the same time the mice were being fed the high fat diet.

A more attractive option was to use the next generation. No DES would be injected, yet this generation has a substantial rate of endometrial cancer somehow related to the fact that their "grandmothers" had been injected with DES. In addition, these mice develop ovarian cancer, which is normally rare in mice. Since ovarian cancer is also linked to international differences in dietary fat, this was an attractive feature. Like most mice, they also get mammary tumors. They have only a low frequency of pituitary tumors. This is an advantage, because if dietary fat affects the hypothalamus, it might show up in the form of more pituitary tumors.

The experiment consisted of putting "DES daughter" mice on diets with 4 different percentages of fat as soon as they became sexually mature. They were bred and kept on their special diets throughout pregnancy, but were changed to a standard diet as soon as their pups were born. The "DES granddaughter" mice were raised to old age and terminal illness. A comparable group of mice without any exposure to DES was also used. The experiment was completed by collecting tumors, studying them under the microscope, and comparing the different groups for an effect of prenatal exposure to high fat.

Cancer from High Fat during Pregnancy

The first difference to show up clearly was that all the large pituitary tumors were in the group exposed to high fat prenatally, regardless of whether or not the mice had a history of exposure to DES. The lack of difference between DES and non-DES mice was not surprising, since only the DES daughter mice would be expected to have a high incidence of pituitary tumors, not the DES granddaughter mice. The next striking effect was on endometrial tumors of the uterus. The DES granddaughter mice were expected to get uterine tumors anyway. However, there were dramatic differences among them, depending on how much fat was in the prenatal diet. With the lower amounts of fat, uterine tumors were rare. With the higher amounts of fat in the maternal diet, there were quite a few endometrial tumors. The mice exposed to the highest amount of fat before birth often developed two such tumors in the same uterus. This type of response, where the amount of cancer increases in proportion to the dose of the cancer-producing agent, is often considered the most convincing proof that the agent under study is responsible for the cancer. In other words, this was a very convincing demonstration that a high fat diet during pregnancy causes cancer in the offspring.

Reproductive Tumors in Control Mice

Glandular types of reproductive tract tumors are rare in mice, including the strain of mice I was using, so I did not expect to see them in the control group. However, a significant number of these tumors did appear in control mice exposed prenatally to high fat. Another unusual finding was that all of the mammary tumor metastases to the lung were in the animals exposed prenatally to high fat, regardless of whether there was ancestral exposure to DES. The spread of tumors to other organs is a very important issue. If breast tumors just stayed in the breast, the surgeon could easily remove them. It is the colonies, or metastases, in other organs that makes cancer a commonly fatal disease. These metastases in mice exposed prenatally to high fat have a parallel in human populations. Breast tumors are more often fatal in America than in Japan - where the diet is low in fat.

Thus, feeding diets high in fat during pregnancy caused the offspring to develop an increased number of endometrial tumors, ovarian tumors, and malignant breast tumors. This matches the epidemiologic data very well, since these tumors correspond to the three types of tumors in women that increase from country to country with increasing levels of fat in the diet.

How Fat Programs Cancer

The induction of pituitary tumors by a high fat diet does not prove that fat acts on the differentiation of the hypothalamus, but it does make this an attractive hypothesis. A feature review article on human breast cancer in a 1988 issue of a major cancer journal reported on the role of endogenous hormones, which are the hormones made in your own body. The authors of this article stated it is virtually certain that endogenous sex hormones play a role in the cause of breast cancer. We already know that disturbing hormone balance in the fetus at the time the hypothalamus is differentiating can upset the functioning of the reproductive system later in life. This includes changing the levels of some endogenous sex hormones. In women, risk factors for reproductive system cancer relate to how this system has been working. If the mother's high fat diet during pregnancy disrupts the differentiation of the fetal hypothalamus, then when that offspring grows up the functioning of its reproductive system will be altered. This is because the functioning of its reproductive system is dependent on the hypothalamus and pituitary gland. Major risk factors for cancer like early menarche, reduced fertility, and late menopause arise from altered function of the reproductive system.

Implications for Human Cancer

Scientists like to find a possible mechanism for any effect they see. This makes it easier to believe that the treatment and outcome represent cause and effect. However, for most people, the important conclusion from the animal study is that the high fat diet during pregnancy definitely did produce cancer. If it does this in mice, it can do the same in people. No one can say that it is not biologically possible for a high fat diet during human pregnancy to cause cancer in the offspring. It is not only possible, it is highly probable that the dramatic differences between female reproductive system cancer in Japan and the U.S. is due largely to differences in diet during pregnancy. The same might be true for the high incidence of prostate cancer in the U.S. compared to Japan. However, male mice were not studied in my experiment due to a shortage of funds. This study should be done eventually, because prostate cancer causes 28,000 deaths every year and there is no effective strategy yet for prevention.

The Stakes

The rate of reproductive system cancer in this country is many times higher than in Japan. Evidence clearly points to an environmental cause. Therefore, reproductive system cancer in America constitutes a massive epidemic which should be stopped. We must not tolerate this epidemic just because it has been around for a long time. If the dietary fat-related cancer rate in the U.S. could be reduced to the level in Japan, consider what it would mean. Out of every six women who would otherwise be destined to develop breast cancer, five would not get the breast cancer. Out of ten women otherwise destined to get uterine cancer, nine would not get this cancer. Out of every four women otherwise destined to get highly lethal ovarian cancer, three would not. Whether controlling dietary fat during pregnancy will really accomplish this large a reduction remains to be seen, but it is a possibility. What a fine heritage to pass on to your daughter!

The Current Generation

What about our children that have already been born? It is too late to protect them from a high fat diet during pregnancy. What about us? Records show that this country was on a high fat diet back when we were born. Is there no way to compensate for this exposure in ourselves and our children who have already been born? The discovery of a dietary fat effect transplacentally (across the placenta from mother to fetus) is too recent for any research to have been done on postnatal preventive measures. However, I did test this possibility with my mouse model of transplacental cancer from DES. I ovariectomized the DES daughter mice (removed their ovaries) and none of the DES types of tumors developed. Of course, this was not intended to be a practical solution, but only a theoretical test. It did prove that this type of transplacentally programmed cancer is not inevitable, but can be prevented. I was unable to raise funds to test for practical methods of prevention.

My experiment with induction of cancer transplacentally by a high fat diet has provided an animal model to test for preventive measures. The first step would be to compare offspring from pregnant mice on low and high fat diets to find out what the fat did to make them different from each other. Specifically, I would try to identify those differences that lead to a higher risk of cancer in one group compared to the other. If this is successful, then postnatal preventive measures could be tested. The need for a new approach to the prevention of reproductive system cancer can be seen in the statistics for breast cancer. Despite the large amount of research on this disease, the number of new cases in the U.S. has not decreased and may even be increasing slightly.

Competition for research funds is very intense. So far, studies on transplacentally induced cancer have not been popular and very little money has been channeled into such studies. Perhaps the revelation that a high fat diet programs for cancer transplacentally will improve accessibility of funds for this type of research.

Critics

I am convinced that a high fat diet during

pregnancy programs human fetuses for cancer later in life. This conclusion is based mainly on one experiment with mice and my interpretation of some of the cancer literature. To draw a striking contrast, the Surgeon General's Report on Nutrition and Health was based on over 2000 scientific papers and was prepared with the help of over 200 scientists. Obviously, my conclusions are much more vulnerable to criticism than the Surgeon General's conclusions. You should give careful consideration to any criticisms raised. The most significant issue in evaluating these criticisms will probably be whether the critics provide a better alternative. If critics reject my conclusion that a high fat diet during pregnancy is dangerous, then what do they recommend? Do they recommend that women continue using the typical high fat American diet? If so, what evidence can they offer that this is safe and will not program your offspring for cancer? Perhaps they will make no recommendation to replace mine, but just criticize. Such an approach abandons the nearly four million women who will become pregnant this year. Despite differences of opinion among scientists, these women will have to decide whether to continue on a high fat diet, or to adopt a reduced fat diet. Advice to wait a few years until more research can be done is useless to them. So listen to the critics, but before abandoning the recommendations in this book, be sure they give you a better alternative. Discuss both sources of information with your physician.

Could Low Fat be Harmful?

Since prenatal development has been disrupted in the past by a variety of agents, it is reasonable to ask whether a low fat diet could have any adverse effects. Certainly the magnitude of fat reduction would be an important issue and extreme reductions should be avoided. Focussing on the general recommendation of reducing fat below 30%, but not going to extremes, there are some obvious points of relevance. The first is that the recommendation of cancer and heart associations and of the surgeon general to reduce dietary fat intake has not excluded women of childbearing age, or even pregnant women. If there were well established risks to the unborn child, surely these agencies would have known about them and issued warnings. Secondly, many women of childbearing age must already have reduced their fat intake below 30% in response to advise from these organizations. Therefore many women have already entered pregnancy on such diets, and will continue to do so. This makes the issue a general one for medicine and not an issue specific to the plan for preventing cancer in the next generation. If any adverse effect is discovered, it should be given wide publicity. Your physician will be able to give you the latest information on this issue. Concerning incidental hazards, such as excessive reduction of protein intake and calories, these problems are addressed in later chapters.

Chapter Three

THE FAT-CONTROLLED DIET

The objective of this chapter is to consider what type of diet would be suitable for use during pregnancy, taking into account the probable danger of high fat. This means a diet that is nutritious enough to support healthy growth of the embryo and fetus, but low enough in fat to avoid programming the fetus for cancer. Starting this diet should not be postponed until pregnancy. There are a variety of reasons for this warning. One reason is the time it takes to adapt the diet plan to your own food preferences. The second is that sometimes pregnancy is well under way before it is diagnosed, and the early part of pregnancy is important for fat control. Also, pregnancy can induce nausea and this would complicate adapting to new food habits. The final reason is speculative at present. It relates to the question of how dietary fat affects the woman's body and eventually the fetus. Does it take time for the body to reverse the effects of a lifetime on a high fat diet? Are hormones already out of balance before pregnancy starts? I do not know the answer, but I believe it is a valid question that we will need to explore through further experimentation. If you are already pregnant, it is certainly worth avoiding further high dietary fat intake. Otherwise, start now to prepare for a possible pregnancy in the future.

Other Diet Plan Books

Book shelves are already warped by the load of low fat diet books. Why do we need another? I investigated that question before taking on the extra work of writing this book. Many low fat diet books were designed for middle-aged men with high cholesterol levels, or other risk factors for cardiovascular disease. The issue of whether such diets would adequately nourish the fetus was not addressed. Other diets were faddish, or extreme and could potentially disrupt fetal development. Some were directed at weight reduction, which should be attended to before pregnancy rather than during pregnancy.

What about books, or chapters especially written for nutrition during pregnancy? Typically, they did not address the issue of high fat. This is understandable, since they were written before the programming of cancer by high fat was discovered. Their advice on nutrition during pregnancy was based on concepts of nutritious foods like whole milk, red meats, cheese and eggs - essentially a disaster from the perspective of programming for cancer. One textbook in our medical library listed specific quantities of specific foods for every pregnant woman to take each day. I calculated the amount of fat in that diet and discovered 49% of the calories came from fat. This amount of fat is higher than the average level in the American diet and as high as the maximum level in my mouse experiment. I cannot criticize the writers of this text, because they were following standard nutritional recommendations existing at the time they wrote the book. Nevertheless, most books or chapters on nutrition for pregnant women need to be re-evaluated in respect to new scientific developments.

Having offered this warning about the potential limitations of other diet books for fetal protection, I can now offer a qualification. If you are already following a low fat plan, it may not be necessary to start on an entirely new diet. Even though a diet book may have been written with emphasis on cardiovascular disease, the diet may be suitable for pregnancy. If the diet has been designed for general health, and avoids radical measures, it may need few, if any changes. The principle objective of my book is to show you how the suitability of your current diet for pregnancy can be evaluated and how it can be corrected, if necessary. This may apply equally well to a diet you have evolved by following the instructions of another diet book. It will depend on whether their diet is sufficiently close to the needs of the fetus and flexible enough to achieve the goals I will describe.

A Lifelong Family Plan

How does the fat-controlled concept for pregnancy relate to dietary recommendations put forth by the American Heart Association, the National Cancer Institute and the Surgeon General's Report on Nutrition and Health? Both organizations and the Surgeon General have urged Americans to reduce the calories obtained from fat to below 30%. The diet plan I will describe for pregnancy also uses the 30% level. This is not a coincidence, because I am looking at the same set of epidemiologic studies that the National Cancer Institute used to reach its conclusions. Thus, a diet suitable for pregnancy can also be good for all family members at all stages of life, with one exception.

The exception is the nursing age baby. Human milk is high in fat, presumably for very good reason. Nursing age babies should be on human milk, as stressed by the Surgeon General's report, or an equivalent substitute with a comparable level of fat. Eventually, when the young child converts to adult foods, a transition to lower fat levels needs to occur. Where the transition should take place is somewhat vague at present and is being debated by pediatricians. The controversy is reflected in the following paragraph from page 573 of the Surgeon General's Report: "The relationship between diet in infancy, childhood, and adolescence and the development of adult atherosclerosis and coronary heart disease is of great current interest. Within the past 5 years, cholesterol-lowering diets for children with elevated blood cholesterol levels (Consensus Development Panel 1985), as well as for those with normal levels (Weidman et al. 1983), have been recommended to prevent onset of the adult disease. These recommendations are that all children older than 2 years adopt a diet that reduces dietary fat intake to 30 percent or less of calories, saturated fat to less than 10% of calories, and daily cholesterol intake to 250 to 300 mg or less. However, other groups have advised against specific recommendations because they find insufficient evidence for the safety and efficacy of such diets in children (AAP Committee on Nutrition 1983c, 1986)."

Does the discovery that fat during pregnancy causes cancer eliminate the need to control fat at other stages of life to prevent cancer? The two are not necessarily mutually exclusive. Certainly the female reproductive system in the fetus is very susceptible to cancer programming by high levels of fat in the mother's diet. There is still the possibility that dietary fat sometime after birth has an effect that adds to the prenatal effect. Secondly, there is evidence that cancer in certain other organs is promoted by high fat diets at other stages of life. Many animal studies have indicated that this is true. Therefore, as far as we know at present, the National Cancer Institute's recommendation that everyone adopt a low fat diet to prevent certain cancers is still valid.

The Hawaiian study mentioned earlier

evaluated saturated fats, unsaturated fats and cholesterol consumption in relation to cancer frequency. It did not seem to make any difference which fat was used. An exception was seen with prostate cancer, which correlated with saturated fats. These measurements were for the culture generally, not for pregnancy specifically. Nevertheless, if the diet was fairly constant for that culture, it was probably representative of what those women ate during pregnancy. The type of fat used in the experiment with pregnant mice was corn oil, which is high in unsaturated fats.

Even though saturated fats are the most dangerous for heart attack, cutting down on fats generally is also recommended. One reason is that the body can synthesize cholesterol anyway. Unless a person has a high cholesterol level and is on a special diet, the fat-controlled diet recommended in this book will be a reasonable step towards lowering risk of heart attack. The one exception to cutting down on fats generally is fish oil. Some intake of fatty fish is recommended for heart attack prevention. The relation of fish oil to cancer is not yet well understood. However, it may be worth having some fish oil in the diet during pregnancy. The reason is that we are using the Japanese diet as a model for a low cancer risk during pregnancy and fish are a standard part of the Japanese diet. Perhaps some fish oil is needed for good fetal development under conditions of a low fat diet. Anyway, it is good for adults and that is sufficient reason for keeping it in the family diet.

A high fat diet is believed to be a factor in obesity. Fat is a concentrated source of energy. In contrast, low fat foods like many vegetables tend to provide bulk with fewer calories. This should help in weight control.

In summary, the recommendation on fats is to reduce fats generally, but include fish oils in the allotment of fat retained in the diet. Optionally, cholesterol and saturated fats could be reduced preferentially as long as the total fat reduction is high enough. Since cholesterol is measured in milligrams and total dietary fat is measured in grams, reducing cholesterol will not contribute noticeably to the percentage of fat reduction.

Thus, if a family is following a fat-controlled diet this will not only benefit a woman preparing for pregnancy, it will benefit all the family members. Everyone will have a better chance to control weight, avoid cancer and avoid heart attack.

Flexibility in Selection of Foods

Many diet books specify which foods to eat for which meals. This has the advantage of simplicity. The reader does not have to decide how to design an appropriate meal. The disadvantage is that you do not get a chance to select your favorite food, or to avoid those that do not agree with you. If you have a whole family to feed, the problem of food preferences becomes much greater. My solution is to show you how to calculate the amount of fat in your diet, so you can select your own foods, recipes and meal combinations.

Approximate or Exact?

One approach to reducing dietary fat is to suggest eating less of the high fat foods and more of the low fat foods. Examples of high fat foods would be red meats and dairy products; low fat foods would be most fruits and vegetables. This method could be used in combination with the first table at the end of this book. The table lists the fat content of a large number of foods. If you use this method how will you know if you have reduced fat intake enough, or even too much? That approach is certainly better than doing nothing to reduce fat. However, is it enough to protect the fetus?

An exact method is needed only if specific limits have to be set. One limit agreed upon is to reduce our intake of fat to below 30% by calories. Maximum reduction has not generally been defined. Animal experimentation would support a very low level of fat intake. However, more information is needed about low fat levels in human pregnancy before considering drastic reductions. The best guide we have at present is the Japanese culture. In the traditional Japanese diet, 20% of their calories come from fat. Since Japanese children develop and grow well, we can assume it is safe to go that low in fat. Therefore, the target we are setting for a fat-controlled diet is to consume between 20% and 30% of calories from fat. This is a relatively wide range. Both international studies and the study with mice indicate a substantial difference in cancer rate could exist between the top and bottom of this range. Dropping from the current average rate of 37% to just below 30% would be a significant accomplishment. Yet, if a person can reach the 20% level, this could be an additional very important achievement.

The next chapter explains a rapid method for controlling fat intake. It will show you how many grams of fat you can safely consume in one meal. Then it will show how to add up the number of fat grams in the food you eat. Chapters Five and Six show a more comprehensive method for diet analysis. However, the recipes and menus in these chapters also provide more practice in using the fast method. Therefore, regardless of whether you finally decide to use the fast method, or the comprehensive method, be sure to read all of the chapters.

Chapter Four

A FAST WAY TO LIMIT FAT INTAKE

A thorough analysis of diet provides insights concerning all the energy-producing components and how to balance them for good nutrition. However, many people will lack the time or the inclination to perform such a detailed analysis. In this chapter, I will describe a shortcut for control of fat intake. In subsequent chapters, the comprehensive method of analysis will be explained. The fast method will allow you to get started now and develop experience with diet control. A decision about whether to expand into the comprehensive method can be made later.

Recommended Caloric Intake

The fast way to control fat intake is based on making an assumption about the total amount of food energy you need each day, as expressed in calories. Table 1 on the next page shows the caloric intake recommended by the National Research Council in 1980. An explanation for each column of the table is given below the table.

TABLE 1. Estimate of calories needed according to age, sex and body size.

Category	Age yrs.	Wt lb	Ht. in.	Energy cal.	Range cal.
Child	1-3	29	35	1300	900-1800
	4-6	44	44	1700	1300-2300
	7-10	62	52	2400	1650-3300
Males	11-14	99	62	2700	2000-3700
	15-18	145	69	2800	2100-3900
	19-22	154	70	2900	2500-3300
	23-50	154	70	2700	2300-3100
	51-75	154	70	2400	2000-2800
Females	11-14	101	62	2200	1500-3000
	15-18	120	64	2100	1200-3000
	19-22	120	64	2100	1700-2500
	23-50	120	64	2000	1600-2400
	51-75	120	64	1800	1400-2200
Pregnancy				+300	
Lactation				+500	

The sex and age categories in the first two columns reflect average differences in energy usage, extra energy demands during growth periods, and decreased energy usage with aging. The next two columns on weight and height show averages for men and women in the designated age ranges. If you do not fit the average, then an adjustment will need to be made for caloric intake. The next column, labelled Energy, shows how many calories you should consume per day, if you are average size with a moderate level of physical activity. The last column shows a range of calorie intake to compensate for differences from the average in body size or exercise. You can make an approximation of your own daily energy usage from this table. A person who is considerably larger than average and has an intensive exercise program, or a physically demanding job, would be at the upper end of the range. For example, a high level of physical activity justifies adding an extra 200 to 300 calories. Another 200 to 300 calories could be added for large body size. Large body size does not include obesity. Obesity comes from an excessively sedentary life, or overeating, or both. In either case, too few calories are being burned relative to food intake and the caloric allotment should be decreased rather than increased. Small body size relative to the stated height and weight listed in the table would justify reducing calories below average, unless activity level was above average. If pregnant, consult Chapter Seven for a discussion of special energy demands and limitation on minimum caloric intake. If you are not sure about being different from average, it is probably better to use the average figure. The number of calories actually consumed in one day can be calculated by keeping track of food intake, as explained in later chapters. However, measuring daily food intake is time-consuming, whereas an estimate from the table will allow you to get started immediately on dietary fat control.

Range of Fat Intake

Since we have already decided that the healthy range of fat intake is 20% to 30% of calories, it is

TABLE 2. Range of fat intake according to daily allotment of calories.

Calories	Fat Intake (grams)	
	daily	per meal
1000	22-33	7-11
1200	27-40	9-13
1400	31-47	10-16
1600	36-53	12-18
1800	40-60	13-20
1900	42-63	14-21
2000	44-67	15-22
2100	47-70	16-23
2200	49-73	16-24
2300	51-77	17-26
2400	53-80	18-27
2500	56-83	19-28
2600	58-87	19-29
2800	62-93	21-31
3000	67-100	22-33
3200	71-107	24-36
3400	76-113	25-38
3600	80-120	27-40
3800	84-127	28-42

easy to calculate the amount of fat allowed per meal. Table 2 above gives examples of recommended daily fat intake. Find your recommended daily caloric intake according to your sex and age from Table 1 on page 44. Find that figure in the first column (labelled Calories) in Table 2 above, then read across. The second column shows your allotment of fat for a complete day. The third column shows how many grams of fat you should eat in a single meal. Both the second and third columns show a range in grams of fat allowed. The range in grams corresponds to our ideal range of fat intake, namely, 20% to 30% of calories consumed. We can explore how these two tables work by using a hypothetical person. From Table 1 we see that an average size woman, in the age range of 23 to 50 and having an average level of activity, would ideally consume 2000 calories per day. From Table 2 we see that her dietary fat allowance would be 44-67 grams per day, or 15-22 grams per meal, assuming three meals a day and no fat-containing snacks. This range will now be used to give examples of how to work with specific meals and limit fat intake to a safe level.

Limiting Fat Intake for One Meal

Suppose you planned to go to a fast-food restaurant for lunch and were planning in advance what to order. Hamburgers have a reputation for being high in fat. Does that rule them out? Look through the sets of tables at the back of this book. There are three sets of tables. The first table shows fat, protein, and carbohydrate content for many foods. This is the only table we are concerned with in this chapter. The other two tables list vitamin content of foods and will be discussed in a later chapter. In the first table, look under Ground beef. Only the columns headed FOOD, MEASURE, and FAT concern us at this time. That part of the table is reproduced below.

FOOD	MEASURE	FAT gm.	FAT %
Ground beef, 10% fat	patty	10	49%
Ground beef, 21% fat	patty	17	66%

Assuming the higher fat beef would be used in a hamburger, follow the line with Ground beef, 21% fat (incidentally, notice that the method for designating percent fat in the FOOD column does not match the method used in the FAT % column. This will be explained in the next chapter.)   The MEASURE column typically lists a single serving, in this case, one 3 oz. patty. The next column shows FAT, gm., in this case 17 grams. Consider the other ingredients of the hamburger. Consult the first table at the back of the book again. It shows that there is no significant amount of fat in tomato ketchup, or mustard, or lettuce, or onion, but the hamburger bun has 2 grams of fat. A conservative teaspoon of mayonnaise would add about 4 grams of fat, so the complete hamburger could have at least 23 grams of fat. Compare the 23 grams of fat in one hamburger with your allotted range of fat for one meal. Using our hypothetical average woman, the range is 15-22 grams.   The hamburger is marginally acceptable if the beef is the only fat-containing item in the meal.   If we include 10 french fries, the food table at the end of the book (see under Potatoes, french fried) shows this adds 7 more grams of fat. The total is now 30 grams, or well above the recommended maximum.   A shake would raise the total to a disastrous 39 grams, or nearly double the recommended maximum of 22 grams.

The Salad Alternative

A prepackaged salad from a fast-food restaurant can be a filling, low fat alternative to the traditional hamburger. In one restaurant's chicken salad, the chicken weighed 2 ounces. Since it was white meat, it should have contained only 2 grams of fat. The other ingredients were vegetables, with no significant fat content. The major determinant of fat content for this salad was the salad dressing. One tablespoon of thousand island dressing adds 8 grams of fat, which would give a total of 10 grams for the salad. This allows 5 to 12 grams for the rest of the meal. However, if the whole package of dressing supplied by the restaurant were poured over the salad it would add 40 grams of fat instead of 8 grams. A similar problem exists at salad bars. The lettuce and most other vegetables are free of fat. However, there are many temptations, like hard boiled egg and cheese shavings, that rapidly add grams of fat. A heaping tablespoon of chopped, hard-boiled egg weighs half an ounce - equivalent to one quarter of an egg - and has 1.5 grams of fat. A heaping tablespoon of grated cheddar cheese, casually scooped up and not packed, weighs a fifth of an ounce and adds about 2 grams of fat.

Fast-Food Literature

Food items from fast-food restaurants can be taken home and weighed to calculate total fat content. A much easier alternative is to use published figures. Some fast-food chains will provide pamphlets of nutritional information about their servings, if asked. Alternatively, books listing nutritional contents of foods from a variety of fast-food restaurants are available. These are very worthwhile for people who eat a lot of their meals at such restaurants. One small book, designed as a guide for diabetics, lists food values for many food chains. Although the emphasis of this book is on calories, it lists the grams of fat for each standard serving. Another book lists fast food as one section in an extensive listing of food values (*Food Values of Portions Commonly Used* by Pennington and Church). Studying such literature reveals some interesting facts. A small hamburger can have as little as 12 grams of fat, whereas cheeseburgers and deluxe hamburgers commonly exceed 30 grams.

Frozen Dinners

The easiest home meal to calculate is the frozen dinner available in grocery stores in the form of a meat and vegetable dinner for one person. Most of these dinners show the composition on the package, including the grams of fat. Thus, the amount of fat in the major part of the meal can be seen at a glance. Fat content can vary widely even when the type of meat is the same. For example, three different chicken dinners, each weighing 10 to 12 ounces, had 10, 18 and 33 grams of fat. Obviously, the one with 33 grams is out of range for one meal. The dinner with 18 grams would be within range, but would not allow much additional fat from other items that might be eaten in addition to the frozen dinner. Since the latter had only 380 calories, additional food would usually be needed to supply enough energy and to be sufficiently filling.

Another convenience food is the family size package of a frozen main course. For example, one brand of beef patties in gravy for four people had a label showing the composition of a single 8 ounce serving. Each person would get 16 grams of fat. Whether this amount of fat is too much would depend on what other foods were eaten with the beef patties. In general, the amount of fat acceptable in a single item like this would be less than in a frozen meal, because the latter usually contains vegetables and sometimes a dessert.

A Low Fat Breakfast

Generally, the easiest meal to analyze and the easiest to keep at a low fat level is breakfast. Most cold or hot cereals contain 0 to 2 grams of fat per serving, as listed on the cereal box. Milk adds 8, 5, 3, or 0 grams of fat for a cup of whole, 2%, 1%, or skim milk, respectively, as listed in the food table at the back of this book. The usual breakfast beverages of orange juice or coffee lack fat, except that a tablespoon of half-and-half or light cream in coffee would add 2 to 3 grams of fat. Toast contributes 1 gram per slice for the bread, 4 grams per teaspoon for margarine or butter, but no fat for jam.   Thus a breakfast of orange juice, a bowl of cereal with half a cup of 2% milk, 2 slices of buttered toast with jam, and coffee with cream adds up to between 15 and 17 grams of fat - a low fat breakfast. Notice that the two teaspoons of butter (8 grams of fat) for toast account for half of the total fat in the meal.

People who like bacon, eggs, and sausage for breakfast have a much greater fat-control problem.   An egg and two slices of bacon total 18 grams of fat.   Two links of pork sausage have 12 grams, while 2 oz. of country style sausage contain 18 grams of fat.   Any one of these dishes would leave almost no leeway for adding any other fat-containing items to the meal.   Breakfast dishes at fast-food restaurants reflect this problem.   Their meat and egg combinations tend to run in the 20 to 40 gram range for fat content.

The Question of Carry-over

Some people have no appetite for breakfast. They may prefer black coffee and a raisin bagel - only 1 gram of fat. Does this mean that the next meal can have double the recommended fat level? Can the 14 to 21 unused grams of fat from breakfast be carried over to lunch for a grand total fat splurge of 29 to 43 grams? I do not know how fat programs the fetus for cancer, so cannot give a scientifically proven answer to this question. However, I would strongly recommend against such a carry-over. If the speculation in Chapter Ten on fatty acids in relation to fetal blood protein and estrogen can be used as a provisional guide, then flooding the fetus with products of fat digestion from a single high fat meal could have an adverse effect. Pending results from further research, my advise is to keep dietary fat levels low at all times and avoid any feast-and-famine behavior.

A complication to an even distribution of fat is that many people do not distribute their calories evenly between three meals. If your breakfast must be small and accounts for very few of your allotted calories, at least try to distribute the remaining calories and fat somewhat evenly between the remaining two meals. If most of the fat consumed is in two meals, it seems prudent to stay close to the 20% level for the daily total, rather than crowding the 30% maximum. In other words, stay close to 44 total grams per day on a 2000 calorie diet, which would not exceed 22 grams of fat per meal even if very few fat calories were consumed at breakfast.

Easy Lunches

Busy people often lack time to mix complicated recipes for a meal and have to rely on packaged foods and fresh foods that are ready to eat. A luncheon consisting of soup, sandwich, crackers and a banana would be easy to prepare. It is also easy to analyze for fat content. Roast turkey breast appears to be a relatively healthy choice for a sliced luncheon meat. Two slices of turkey can be combined with tomato and lettuce on whole wheat bread spread with light mayonnaise. Fat content of the turkey and light mayonnaise is on the package label and the other ingredients of the meal can be found in the food table at the back of this book. Quantities from these sources have to be converted to the quantities used in the meal, so a clear way to keep track is to list the foods and the basic quantities, then use another set of columns to list the amount of food actually eaten and to calculate the fat consumed. The table on the next page shows this calculation. The first two sets of figures are for the measurement units listed on the package, or in the food table, and the number of grams of fat in that size of serving. The second two sets of figures are for the quantities used in the meal and the grams of fat calculated according to whether the quantity used was greater, less, or the same as on the package label, or in the table.

The total fat of 15 grams in this meal is ideal. The calories correspond to one third of the daily allotment for the average woman, so the amount of energy in the meal should be sufficient. If additional fluid is needed, either water or fruit juice could be added without increasing fat content. Alternatively, milk with a lower percentage of fat could replace the 2% milk.

FOOD	FOOD TABLE		MEAL	
	AMOUNT	FAT	AMOUNT	FAT
Soup:				
Vegetable beef	1 cup	2	1 cup	2
Sandwich:				
Wheat bread	1 slice	1	2 slices	2
Turkey	1 slice	1	2 slices	2
Light mayonnaise	1 tbsp	5	2 tsp	3
Fresh tomato	1	0	1/2	0
Romaine lettuce	1 cup	0	2 leaves	0
Beverage:				
Milk, 2%	1 cup	5	1 cup	5
Dessert:				
Graham crackers	2	1	2	1
Banana	1	0	1	0
TOTAL FAT GRAMS IN MEAL:				15

The first time you analyze one of your own meals is the best time to start a record book. If calculations are made on scraps of paper, they are ususlly gone later if you want to refer back to them. Our eating habits are sufficiently repetitive to justify keeping a record of every meal analyzed. A loose leaf notebook is a good selection because it allows for discarding, recopying, rearranging and indexing.

The Complexities of Dinner

Complex recipes and multicourse meals provide a considerable challenge. This is especially true of fancy restaurants where recipes are elaborate and published data are not available. The best defense is experience with home meals. Even a person who does no cooking can browse through cookbooks and find out what high fat ingredients are used in various standard dishes. Rough estimates are better than no awareness of which food combinations are likely to be high in fat. Yet, specific calculations can be made easily when the recipe is available. Current cookbooks often provide information on the fat content of their recipes in response to public concern about reducing fat intake to prevent heart attacks. Note that the content of cholesterol cannot be used as a guide to total fat content. Cholesterol is measured in milligrams, and a milligram is only one thousandth of a gram.

If the recipe does not list fat content, just identify the fat-containing ingredients, add up the total and divide by number of servings. Generally, vegetables, fruits, and grains do not add significant fat. Some exceptions are avocados, nuts, and olives. Meats, cooking oils, eggs and dairy products are common sources of fat in recipes. A dish made by cooking beef and vegetables together would typically have margarine or cooking oil as the main fatty ingredient in addition to the meat. Beef could contribute anywhere from 7 to 33 grams of fat, depending on the type of beef (see entries under Beef in the table at the back of this book). If the recipe calls for 2 tablespoons of safflower oil (28 grams of fat) and serves four, add 7 grams of fat to the 7-33 grams from the beef. Whether this dish will be sufficiently low in fat depends heavily on whether the cut of meat used is low or high in fat. It also depends on whether you consume 3 oz. of beef, as listed in the table as a serving size for the fat content specified, or a larger serving, which would add additional grams of fat. The next step would be to add in the fat content of the other courses.

Fat Content of a Dinner

A complete, traditional dinner is somewhat more time-consuming to analyze than a luncheon, but not any more difficult unless there are complicated recipes involved. Consider a dinner of fruit salad, roast chicken, vegetables, and a mixed gelatin-fruit-ice cream dessert. The basic technique is to seek out the fat-containing items. In this meal, most of the fat is in the flavoring and dessert. For example, the sour cream for the baked potato, the margarine for the beans and corn, the half-and-half in the coffee, and the ice cream in the dessert recipe account for 13 of the 17 grams of fat in this meal, as listed in the next table. As with the luncheon listing just presented, the table of dinner contents on the next page shows the food item in the first column, the standard measurements from the food table in the second and third columns, and the specific figures for the meal in the last two columns. Although there is no fat in the fruit salad, the baked potato, and the beans, they are listed to provide a full view of the menu. The fruit salad is a mixture of fresh fruits, none of which had any fat, as confirmed by looking up each component fruit individually. Each serving of chicken was 2 ounces divided equally between dark and white meat. The gelatin-fruit-ice cream dessert was from a recipe found on a gelatin dessert package. Since the gelatin and diced fruit in the recipe lacked fat, only the ice cream content had to be calculated. The recipe required one quart of ice cream and served 12 people, so each person received the equivalent of just under 3 ounces of ice cream. All the calculations in the table are rounded off to the nearest whole number. The fat in this full course dinner is near the desirable lower end of the 15-22 gram range. Yet, the total energy is more than a third of the 2000 calorie daily quota. This compensates for breakfast, which is usually below a third of the daily caloric quota.

FOOD	FOOD TABLE		MEAL	
	AMOUNT	FAT	AMOUNT	FAT
Fruit salad	1 cup	0	1 cup	0
Chicken, dark	1 oz	2	1 oz	2
Chicken, light	1 oz	1	1 oz	1
Baked potato	1	0	1	0
Sour cream	1 cup	48	1 tbsp	3
Green beans	1 cup	0	1 cup	0
Margarine	1 tbsp	12	1/4 tsp	1
Corn, fresh	1 ear	1	1 ear	1
Margarine	1 tbsp	12	1/2 tsp	2
Ice cream	1 cup	14	3 oz.	5
Half & half	1 cup	28	1 tbsp	2
TOTAL FAT GRAMS IN MEAL:				17

A Lifetime of Measuring?

The combination of analyzing the main course recipe for fat content and then having to check all the other items in the meal may seem overwhelming, especially if this has to be done every day for every meal. The solution comes from the extensive repetition in most people's diet. Once a recipe is analyzed, the fat content per serving can be written next to the recipe. Similarly, once a standard meal combination is confirmed to fall within the specified range of fat content, it does not need to be rechecked each time it is used. Experience gained in calculations will provide sophistication in recognizing high and low fat foods. Usually, one vegetable can be substituted for another, unless the cooking method changes to add more of some high fat ingredient like butter. Fruits for dessert can be varied without requiring extra calculations. A person's beverage tends to remain constant, so 2-3 grams for coffee cream is soon added in without having to look it up. Just get started and gain some experience. Concentrate on one meal at a time. You'll be surprised how simple it becomes after a week or two.

Recognizing Fatty Foods

One way to get started on fat reduction is to look through the first table on food values at the end of the book and notice which foods are high or low in fat. The column labelled FAT, GRAMS shows the grams of fat in one serving and can be used for comparison with your ideal range of fat per meal.   However, some of the measures are intended for recipes rather than individual consumption, like one cup of corn oil. Another way to use the table is to work with percent fat. The next column, labelled FAT, % can be used for comparison against the standard recommendation to get less than 30% of calories from fat. Any food with a figure higher than 30% in this column will tend to increase your fat intake above the recommended level.   Similarly, foods with a number below 30% will help to compensate for the high fat foods.

The Most Difficult Problem

The real problem is not the calculations, it is the changing of eating habits.   If a person overeats, or has a strong preference for high fat foods, or both, this will be the most difficult problem to solve.   Multiple servings of dishes with moderate fat content can build up total fat intake to unsafe levels.   An emergency measure for excessive appetite is to take small servings of fatty foods and fill up on fat-free foods.   The basic issue of balancing caloric intake and caloric expenditure is discussed later in this book. Switching from high fat foods to low fat foods requires awareness of the problem and a willingness to experiment.   Again, plunge in and see what happens.   The way to develop an appreciation of flavors other than those arising from high fat content is to get used to the other flavors. This works best when combined with caloric restriction. A good appetite is the ideal starting point for enjoying foods low in fat and sugar.

Practice in Diet Analysis

The next two chapters focus on a more comprehensive method of diet analysis. Nevertheless, recipes and menus listed in the comprehensive tables that start about half way through Chapter Five can be used to practice the fast method. If you are not interested in the comprehensive method, just ignore the columns labelled PROT, CARBO, and CAL. Use only the columns labelled FOOD, AMT and FAT. In the two lines across the bottom of each table, just pick out the TOTALS line, read the total grams of fat, and see how high this is compared to your goal for an optimal intake of fat in one meal.

Fast Method for Protein

Anticipating pregnancy, it will be necessary eventually to deal with the protein content of meals. For this reason alone, it is important to study the next two chapters. Yet, it is still possible to avoid the full range of calculations shown in Chapters Five and Six. Protein could be calculated the same way as was shown for fat in this chapter. Chapters Five and Seven both set goals for daily intake of protein in grams. Therefore, a shortcut would be to add up the number of grams of protein in each meal in the same way as adding up fat. For an average woman, the goal would be 44 grams of protein per day when not pregnant and 74 grams of protein per day during pregnancy. The single meal equivalent would be 15 grams when not pregnant and 25 grams during pregnancy. As far as I know, an even distribution of protein between meals is not a big issue, in contrast to fat. However, a moderately good distribution between meals seems like a reasonable idea. A moderate excess is also not an issue, but a very large excess might be.

Examples of Protein Calculation

In the breakfast listed earlier under "A Low Fat Breakfast" the protein content can be added up using food values from the table at the end of this book and from the cereal box. Listing just the food items containing protein, the protein content was 6 grams from the cereal with milk, and 6 grams from the 2 slices of wheat toast. Thus, the total protein in this low fat breakfast was 12 grams. This is a reasonable approximation of the recommended 15 grams per meal for a non-pregnant woman, especially since breakfast is usually lower in protein than other meals of the day. The protein content could be increased for pregnancy by adding a 1 ounce serving of a special high protein dry cereal. With half a cup of 2%

milk on the cereal, this would increase the protein content by 10 grams to a new total of 24 grams, which is comparable to the recommended 25 grams per meal. Of course, when an additional item is added to the meal, the effect on fat content must also be checked. The extra 2 grams of fat from the half cup of 2% milk would result in 17 to 19 total grams of fat and so would not exceed the 22 gram maximum. Alternatively, a lower fat milk could be used. An additional advantage of the extra bowl of cereal is the added calcium from the milk, as well as the extra vitamins and minerals from the fortified cereal.

A similar protein calculation for the sandwich meal listed under "Easy Lunches" is equally simple. Again we will find the protein content from the food table and from the package of turkey meat, and will list only foods with significant protein content. The protein content was 5 grams from vegetable beef soup, 6 grams from wheat bread, 12 grams from two slices of turkey, 1 gram from tomato and lettuce, 8 grams from the glass of milk, 1 gram from the graham crackers and 1 gram from the banana. The total protein content of that light luncheon was 34 grams, which is most of the recommended 44 grams a day for the non-pregnant woman and almost half the total day's quota of 74 grams for a pregnant woman.

The procedure for checking protein intake by this rapid method is not different from checking fat intake, except for the differences in the recommended totals. Both could be done at the same time by just adding an extra column for protein in the tables shown earlier in this chapter. The extra work is well worth the effort, both for the individual and in planning meals for the whole family.

Chapter Five

A COMPLETE DIETARY ANALYSIS METHOD

A complete analysis of all energy-producing components of the diet provides additional insight on developing good nutritional habits.   One specific advantage is that total caloric intake can be determined accurately.   A second advantage is that the balance of nutrients can be checked. The method does require more written notations and calculations than the fast method of the previous chapter.   A decision as to whether to use this method depends on interest and available time. Even if you decide not to use the method, reading through this chapter and Chapter Six could help in using the fast method.

How to Calculate Percent Fat by Calories

The three food categories that produce energy in normal foods are protein, carbohydrate and fat. Alcohol also adds calories, as can be seen by looking up alcoholic drinks in the food table (e.g., Whisky).   The percent of calories derived from fat is calculated by multiplying the grams of fat by 9

	1 OUNCE CEREAL	WITH 1/2 CUP SKIM MILK
CALORIES	110	150
PROTEIN	4 g	8 g
CARBOHYDRATE	20 g	26 g
FAT	2 g	2 g

and dividing this number by the total calories in the food serving. For example, a typical box of dry cereal will have information listed on its side similar to what is shown in the table above. Other ingredients like vitamins and minerals are listed, but we only need the figures given above for calculations on percentage of fat. Since both calories and fat are known, calculation of percent calories from fat is very simple. The 2 grams of fat are multiplied by 9, so 18 calories out of the 110 calories for cereal are derived from fat. Dividing 18 fat calories by 110 total calories gives 0.16, or 16%. So the cereal has 16% of its calories derived from fat. Many cereals list 0 grams of fat, which is automatically 0% fat without any calculation. The dish of cereal complete with skim milk still only has 2 grams of fat, but the total calories have risen to 150. This time, the 18 fat calories are divided by 150 total calories and this equals only 12% fat in the mixture of cereal and skim milk. If the label had not given total calories, they could have been calculated from the ingredients. The 4 grams of protein and 20 grams of carbohydrate are both multiplied by 4, giving a subtotal of 96 calories. Add the 18 calories from fat for a total of 114 calories. This is a reasonable approximation of the 110 calories shown on the package. The reason for the difference of 4 calories is that the company used a more exact method to determine the number of calories in their product.

Using the Percent Fat Method for Food Selection

Casually scanning the labels in the grocery store can often provide an estimate of degree of fat by mental arithmetic. For example, the label on a can of soup shows for protein, carbohydrate and fat, 1 gram, 6 grams and 2 grams in a 4 ounce serving and a total of 50 calories. Mentally, this is 2 times 9, or 18 calories from fat out of 50, which is the same as 36 out of 100, or 36%. Instructions for serving the soup specify mixing with an equal amount of water. This does not change the percentage of fat and can be ignored when calculating fat in the diet.

For those of us not enthused about mental arithmetic, a simple pocket calculator is a great convenience. They are available for under $10. To use a calculator for the soup label described above, enter 2 x 9 = 18 then divide by 50 to find percent fat by calories.

Would the soup be unuseable for our diet, since it exceeded our target range? Not necessarily, since this would depend on how much soup was consumed and what other foods were eaten in the same meal. Foods are mixed together in the stomach and broken down into basic chemical

FOOD	AMT	PROT	CARBO	FAT	CAL
Cereal	1 oz	4	20	2	110
Milk, skim	1/2 cup	4	6	0	40
Soup concentrate	4 oz	1	6	2	50
TOTALS		9	32	4	200

(Abbreviations in table: AMT = amount of serving, PROT = protein, CARBO = carbohydrate, CAL = calories.)

fragments by the digestive enzymes, so it is reasonable to assume that what counts is the total amount of fat in the meal. Suppose a person consumed 1 ounce of cereal with a 1/2 cup of skim milk and also 4 ounces of the soup (disregarding the fact that this is a highly improbable combination). The table above summarizes the values from the cereal box and soup can.

Total calories from fat are 4 x 9 = 36 calories. Divided by 200, this comes to 18% fat, which is well below the maximum of 30%. The total fat is low, so the fact that the soup by itself was a little high in fat is not a problem.

The reasoning for combining foods in one meal does not apply to combining all the meals of one day. As mentioned in the last chapter, a high fat meal would send a mass of fat into the circulation at one time. Unless evidence can be produced to the contrary, it would be safer to assume this is dangerous for the fetus. Therefore, the plan recommended here will be based on holding each meal in the 20% to 30% range. This is not to propose that one or two percentage points would make a difference. The proposal is to reject the assumption that breakfast at 10% fat would compensate for a 40% fat dinner.

Many foods in the grocery store do not have labels showing composition. Meats, fresh fruits and vegetables will not have such labels. The answer is to familiarize yourself with the values in the table on percent fat at the end of this book. The calculations of percent fat were made by converting grams to calories, rather than as a proportion of the column on total calories. The calculations were performed in this manner so that the individual percentages would add up to 100%. Skimming through the tables will illustrate that most meats, nuts, dairy products, cakes and cookies are high in fat; fruits and vegetables are almost all low in fat. There are exceptions, like avocados with 82% fat. Oils, butter, margarine, lard are 100% fat and even small amounts can have a dramatic impact on percent of fat in a meal, as will be illustrated later.

One type of food labelling can be confusing. For example, a packaged turkey product had a label claiming 15% fat content. However, the label also listed the contents of one serving as 4 grams of fat and a total of 60 calories. Fat calories would be 9 x 4 = 36 calories. This is 60% of total calories. The reason for the label showing 15% fat instead of 60% fat is that the company used a different method of calculation and was not basing their claim on percent of calories. Their method was the same as used for the ground beef listed in

CATEGORY	AGE (years)	WEIGHT (pounds)	HEIGHT (inches)	PROTEIN (grams)
Children	1-3	29	35	23
	4-6	44	44	30
	7-10	62	52	34
Males	11-14	99	62	45
	15-18	145	69	56
	19-22	154	70	56
	23-50	154	70	56
	51 +	154	70	56
Females	11-14	101	62	46
	15-18	120	64	46
	19-22	120	64	44
	23-50	120	64	44
	51 +	120	64	44
Pregnant				+30
Lactating				+20

Chapter Four and in the food table, where "Ground Beef, 21%" turns out to have 66% fat by calories.

Reasons for Listing Protein

Protein is not needed for calculating percent fat unless total calories are not listed - a rare occurrence. Also, the average American diet is high in protein, so a deficiency is unlikely. However, the average American diet carries a high risk for cancer and heart attack. The latter are blamed on high fat, but a major source of fat is meat, which is high in protein. Reducing fat in most diets will mean reducing protein also.

Therefore, it is logical to keep track of protein while changing your diet. The National Research Council made specific recommendations in 1980 for daily intake of protein. These recommendations are shown in the table on the preceeding page (page 70). Notice that the requirement for protein stays constant during the adult period. Differences in protein requirement between family members will be balanced by differences in food intake, as can be seen by referring back to the table on recommended caloric intake in Chapter Four. If your meal calculations show that you are consuming the recommended amount of calories and protein, then the same should be true for others whose volume of food eaten is also based on the recommended number of calories. An exception to this is the decrease of calories with aging without a corresponding decrease in protein requirement. Nevertheless, protein intake will probably be above the recommended minimum, as will be seen in the examples given on the following pages, so a need for supplementing their diet is unlikely.

Reasons for Listing Carbohydrate

There is no recommended daily dietary allowance for carbohydrate. Yet, it is an important part of the diet. The reason is that it is needed as the major source of energy. Fat must be reduced as a source of energy. If protein were increased to make up the energy difference, then the consumption of protein would be too high. To achieve a proper dietary balance, carbohydrate should be increased. For optimal health, most of the carbohydrate should be in the form of complex carbohydrates, not simple sugars like sucrose (table sugar). In the examples of meals and recipes that will be given, the percent of calories derived from carbohydrate will be listed. Then it will be easy to see whether carbohydrate is the major source of energy, as recommended.

How to Calculate Fat in a Simple Meal

The easiest meal to analyze for most people will be breakfast. To illustrate the problem with some American eating habits, I will first list a high fat breakfast. In the headings for the table, AMT = amount of food used, PROT = protein, CARBO = carbohydrate. The amounts of protein, etc. are in grams. The line labelled "% of calories" was derived by multiplying the grams of protein and carbohydrate by 4 and the fat by 9. These totals were then added and divided into the totals for each food component to get the individual percentages. If you are not interested in the percentages for protein and carbohydrate, the fat percentage can be derived from an easier calculation. Just multiply the fat grams by 9 and divide this by the total calories listed at the bottom of the last column. The result may be slightly different from the percentage given in the table, because the calorie column was derived by a more accurate method than multiplying the approximate grams of individual components by

FOOD	AMT	PROT	CARBO	FAT	CAL
Orange juice	1 cup	2	29	0	120
Eggs	2	12	2	12	160
Bacon	2 slices	4	0	8	85
Toast	2 slices	6	28	2	130
Margarine	1 tbsp	0	0	12	100
Jam	1 tbsp	0	14	0	55
Coffee	1 cup	0	0	0	0
Cream	1 tbsp	0	1	3	30
TOTALS		24	74	37	680
% of calories		13%	41%	46%	

their caloric value.

The amount of protein in the breakfast shown above is unnecessarily high. Using the daily recommended level of 44 grams for an average woman, this is half the day's allotment. Carbohydrate is deficient in contributing less than half the total calories. The real problem lies with the fat. The 46% of calories coming from fat is double the amount recommended. This deficiency would also be quickly recognized by the fast method of Chapter Four. To use the above table for the fast method of Chapter Four, just ignore the columns labelled PROT, CARBO and CAL. If you were constructing a table of your own, you would have three headings: FOOD, AMT and FAT. The only total needed would come from adding up the grams of fat in the FAT column. The 37 total grams of fat in this breakfast is far above the 15 to 22 grams per meal recommended for the average woman. (It would still be on the

FOOD	AMT	PROT	CARBO	FAT	CAL
Grapefruit	1/2	1	13	0	50
Sugar	2 tsp	0	8	0	30
Dry cereal	3/4 cup	2	15	1	85
Skim milk	1 cup	8	12	0	85
Cooked egg	1	6	1	6	80
Toast	1 slice	3	14	1	65
Margarine	1 tsp	0	0	4	33
Marmalade	1 tsp	0	5	0	20
Coffee	1 cup	0	0	0	0
TOTALS		20	68	12	448
% from calories		17%	59%	24%	

chart for someone consuming 3400 calories per day, or more, but then this breakfast would only provide 680 calories instead of the expected 1130 calories.)   In contrast, consider the breakfast in the table above, which was listed in a publication recommending a low fat diet. This is a low fat breakfast, as claimed, with the 24% of calories from fat being in the middle of the 20% to 30% range. Similarly, by the fast method, the 12 grams of fat does not exceed the 15 to 22 grams recommended for our hypothetical average woman. Although eggs are an inexpensive source of good protein, the yolk is a problem. It contains the maximum amount of cholesterol allowed for a whole day, so people watching their intake of cholesterol would probably want to delete the egg. Others may not find the selection of foods to their liking, or the amount of food consistent with their appetite. The obvious next step is to plan a breakfast that will meet your specific needs.

Designing your own breakfast

Most of the information needed to construct a table like the one on the opposite page will be found on food labels, or in the table at the back of this book. One difference can be the serving sizes. You may use different serving sizes from those listed in the tables, or else not be sure what serving sizes you are using. Measurements can be made easily. The only equipment needed is a measuring cup, measuring spoons, and a scale. A simple dietetic scale can be purchased for $10 and a more accurate scale for less than $20. Measurement conversions are listed at the back of the book on the page before the set of food tables. Take a relaxed weekend morning and measure what you are currently eating for breakfast, calculate the percentage of fat and make some adjustments in the menu, if necessary.

Reasons for Listing Calories

The fast method in Chapter Four was based on average caloric needs. Your specific needs may not match the averages. Total caloric intake per day can be derived from adding up three typical meals. If the total is different from your original assumption, you can calculate a new set of figures for the amount of fat to allow yourself. Multiply the new figures for total calories by 20% and 30%. This tells you how many of your total calories can be derived from fat. Divide both of these numbers by 9 to find the range of fat grams allowed per day.

Then divide by three to get the range for each meal.

Listing calories can be useful if your weight is in a steady state and you want to change your menu. If you keep the calories the same, your weight will stay the same. Alternatively, you may wish to decrease your weight. One way to do this is to delete some calories from the meal by removing food items, or reducing serving sizes, while continuing to maintain a good balance of protein, carbohydrate and fat. A weight reduction program should always be accompanied by exercise to help burn off fat and to prevent muscle loss. The amount of fat to lose can be determined best by the use of skinfold calipers. These are simple instruments and the plastic versions can be purchased for $15 to $20. The technique is to pinch up a fold of skin on several parts of the body and measure the fold with the calipers. Tables provided with the instrument list the percentage of body weight that consists of fat, according to your own skinfold thickness. Recommended body fat levels for men range from 14% to 18% and for women from 18% to 24%. When this range is reached, caloric intake should be increased just enough to maintain this level of body fat. However, before selecting a body fat level, be sure to read "Fertility and Body Fat" in Chapter Eight.

Cooking Methods

If food is cooked in fat, or oil, it is likely to

absorb significant amounts and this can have a dramatic effect on the fat content of the cooked food. Using the table on fat content at the back of this book, compare the percent fat for various methods of cooking potatoes. Looking under the word "potato", the fat content ranges from 0% for baking to 44% for frying. Similarly, look up "fish sticks." Although most fish are low in fat, deep fried fish sticks are 49% fat. This fat is not the desirable fish fat, but only the vegetable or meat fat used for cooking. Obviously, it is futile to add fish to the menu for its low fat content and then eat it soaked in cooking oil.

The National Cancer Institute recommends against cooking methods that add carcinogens to meat, like barbecuing, charcoal-broiling, grilling, smoking and frying at high temperatures. There is no evidence, so far, that food cooked in this manner and consumed by pregnant women has led to cancer in the offspring. However, the same compounds (polycyclic aromatic hydrocarbons) have been given to pregnant animals and have caused increased cancer in the offspring. It would be prudent to avoid these cooking methods during pregnancy. There are many other options such as baking, roasting, oven-broiling, microwave cooking, boiling, steaming, poaching, and stewing. Avoidance of cooking methods that add carcinogens need not be limited to pregnancy.

Chapter Six

FAT CONTENT OF MIXTURES AND RECIPES

More complex meals can be calculated the same way as shown for breakfast in the last chapter. It helps if mixtures and recipes are explored ahead of time and selected, or adjusted to conform to the proposed fat level before being incorporated into a total meal calculation. For example, if you use salads frequently it is worth analyzing them for fat content and then adjusting the ingredients if the salad is excessively high in fat. Then when it is added to the full meal, you will not have to find other low fat foods to compensate for a high fat salad. For example:

FOOD	AMT	PROT	CARBO	FAT	CAL
Romaine lettuce	1/2 cup	0.5	1	0	5
Dressing	1 tsp	0	1	2.5	22
Bean sprouts	1/8 cup	0.5	0.9	0	5
Sliced tomatoes	4 oz	1	6	0	28
Croutons	0.5 oz	1.8	8	0.5	44
TOTALS		3.8	16.9	3.0	104
% of calories		14%	61%	25%	

Percent of fat in this salad is in the middle of the recommended range. Also, the 3 grams of fat is a small proportion of the fat quota for one meal. Notice that the lettuce has a lot of bulk, but only adds 1.5 grams of energy producing food, whereas the very small volume of salad dressing adds 3.5 grams. If a tablespoon of dressing had been used instead of a teaspoon, the salad would have been 48% fat. Obviously, salad dressing should not just be dumped on - it should be measured. Lettuce and bean sprouts add a lot of bulk, but it is mostly water. Notice that the few croutons add the greatest amount of carbohydrate and calories. Yet, they are low in fat, although mainly because they are homemade. Vegetarians cannot assume their diet is low in fat. If they fry in oil, or add margarine, salad dressings and sauces, they can rapidly convert their diet to high fat. So they have to calculate the percent fat like everyone else. There is indication that the international differences in cancer rates are linked more to animal fats than to vegetable fats. However, it is too soon to rely on this possibility, especially since the animal experiment on high fat diet during pregnancy was done with vegetable fat.

Cookbook Recipes

Recipes may be easy, or time-consuming to work with, depending on whether the recipe book provides food values. A recently published cookbook (*Weight Watchers Favorite Recipes*) lists the total amount of protein, carbohydrate, fat and calories in each recipe. This is the ideal situation, because the grams of fat can be read at a glance and the percent fat can be calculated immediately. To calculate percent fat, multiply the grams of fat by 9 and divide this number by the total calories. If the recipe is selected for a meal, the figures can be added directly to the other food values for that meal. Another book shows total protein, fat and calories, but leaves out the carbohydrate. For example, one of the dessert recipes lists 5 grams of protein, 2 grams of fat and 185 calories. The percent fat is easily calculated, since the 2 grams of fat represent 2 x 9 = 18 calories out of 185 total calories, which is 10% fat. However, if this recipe was to be added to a total meal analysis, then either the carbohydrate component would have to be left out, or else calculated. To do the latter, the first step is to find the number of calories attributable to fat and protein, which is 18 calories for fat, as derived above. The 5 grams of protein multiplied by 4 gives 20 calories for protein. Since fat and protein account for 38 of the total 185 calories, then carbohydrate accounts for the remaining 147 calories. At 4 calories per gram, the carbohydrate content of this recipe is 147 divided by 4, or 37 grams.

Recipes with No Food Values Listed

If food values are not given for a recipe, the only way to assess its fat content and add the ingredients for a total meal calculation is to list the individual components as we did with

FOOD	AMT	PROT	CARBO	FAT	CAL
Spaghetti, dry	5 oz	20	105	2.5	525
Parmesan cheese	1/3 cup	14	1.3	10	152
Pimiento	1/4 cup	0.5	3.5	0.3	15
Turkey, white	12 oz	112	0	12	600
Flour	1/4 cup	3	22	0.3	105
Onion soup mix	1 pkg	1	6	1	35
Milk, whole	1 cup	8	11	8	150
Peas, cooked	1/2 cup	4	10	0	55
TOTALS (4 servings)		163	159	34	1637
One serving		41	40	9	409
% of calories		40%	40%	20%	

breakfasts in the previous chapter. Due to the work involved, it is best to start with major dishes used frequently. An appropriate recipe for a low fat diet with adequate protein is a poultry tetrazini recipe that can be used for leftover turkey, or chicken. The recipe and its food values are shown in the table above. The single serving is listed to be added to a total meal calculation. The percent fat is low, falling at the bottom of the 20% to 30% range. This is a tasty way of adding a lot of protein to a meal without adding a lot of fat. Notice that the cheese, which by itself is 59% fat, and whole milk, which is 49% fat can be used because they are compensated by the spaghetti, which is almost free of fat. The 9 grams of fat is below the average 15-22 gram target range, so other fat-containing items can be added to the meal.

FOOD	AMT	PROT	CARBO	FAT	CAL
Salad	1 bowl	3.8	16.9	3	104
Tetrazini	1 serving	41	40	9	409
Hawaiian bread	2 oz	4	28	4	172
Cherries	10	1	12	0	45
Water	14 oz	0	0	0	0
TOTALS		50	97	16	730
% of calories		27%	53%	20%	

Adding Recipe Totals to a Meal

The next step is to add the mixture and the recipe to the other foods of a complete dinner. The table above shows the total figures for the salad and the tetrazini, which are then listed with bread, dessert and beverage. The fat content of this meal is low. Since we knew in advance that the salad was 25% fat, the tetrazini was 20% fat, the cherries were 0% fat, the result had to be close to the 20% to 30% range. A quick mental check on the bread would show 36 calories from fat in the total of 172 calories, or 21% fat. Therefore, the whole dinner menu would have to be in the low fat range. We could recognize that even without making the listing and calculations of the above table. This is not an exception. After calculating a number of recipes and meals it becomes fairly easy to recognize low and high fat meals. If your eating habits are fairly repetitive, most of the calculations come in the first few weeks. After that, only the occasional new recipe needs to be mathematically checked. The same is true of protein content. Assuming this is the main protein meal of the day, the 50 grams of protein per person assures adequate daily protein intake, since the other two meals inevitably contain some protein also. If you are following only fat intake, the 16 grams of fat falls at the low end of the range for one meal, and this is optimal.

Substitutions and Deletions

The next issue is substitutions, or deletions when a calculation shows excessive fat content. Some people like to add canned chow mein noodles to a salad. If 1/4 of a cup were added to the salad listed above, it would increase the fat content by 3 grams, raising the total amount of fat in the salad to 6 grams and the percentage of fat to 39%. Obviously the noodles should either be used in very small quantities, or bypassed entirely.

Modifying Recipes

Recipes in which the major source of flavor is a high fat ingredient pose a special problem. An example is a recipe for tuna salad made with a packaged mixture of macaroni and vegetables. The original recipe on the commercial food package for 5 servings recommended adding the contents of the package to 3/4 cup mayonnaise and one can of tuna, without specifying the type of tuna. Using tuna packed in water, the percent fat can be calculated from the following table.

FOOD	AMT	PROT	CARBO	FAT	CAL
Salad mix	1 package	25	140	5	700
Mayonnaise	3/4 cup	0	0	132	1200
Tuna in water	6 1/2 oz	39	0	3	195
TOTALS (5 servings)		64	140	140	2095
One serving		12.8	28	28	424
% of calories		12%	27%	61%	

Percent fat in this recipe is much too high for a main course. Since one serving would have 28 grams of fat, this high fat level could not be balanced with low fat foods in the same meal. For someone on 2000 calories per day, the 28 grams would exceed the meal quota of 15-22 grams established in Chapter Four. If the tuna salad were substituted for the tetrazini in the last meal, this would be the result:

FOOD	AMT	PROT	CARBO	FAT	CAL
Salad	1 bowl	3.8	16.9	2.5	104
Tuna salad	1 serving	12.8	28	28	424
Hawaiian bread	2 oz	4	28	4	172
Cherries	10	1	12	0	45
TOTALS		21.6	85	34.5	745
% of calories		12%	46%	42%	

The fat in this meal is much too high, either by the criterion of 42% fat, or by the content of 34.5 grams. We can propose a modification of the recipe by replacing the regular mayonnaise with a light mayonnaise salad dressing and vanilla yogurt.

Here is the result:

FOOD	AMT	PROT	CARBO	FAT	CAL
Salad mix	1 package	25	140	5	700
Light mayonnaise	3/8 cup	0	6	30	300
Vanilla yogurt	3/8 cup	4	13	1	75
Tuna in water	6 1/2 oz	39	0	3	195
TOTALS (5 servings)		64	159	39	1270
One serving		12.8	32	7.8	254
% of calories		21%	51%	28%	

This modification reduces the fat from 61% to 28%. Since the recipe now has only 7.8 grams of fat, there is plenty of leeway to add other fat-containing dishes to the meal. Consider the meal previously listed, but now with the lower fat tuna salad:

FOOD	AMT	PROT	CARBO	FAT	CAL
Salad	1 bowl	3.8	16.9	2.5	104
Light tuna salad	1 serving	12.8	32	7.8	254
Hawaiian bread	2 oz	4	28	4	172
Cherries	10	1	12	0	45
TOTALS		21.6	89	14.3	575
% of calories		15%	62%	23%	

The percent fat with the modified tuna salad is within the specified range and the number of fat grams is at the lower limit for a 2000 calorie diet. Thus the total meal is satisfactory. I am not claiming that the modified recipe is just as delicious as the original, but it is much healthier.

Recipe Modification with the Fast Method

Notice that in all these meal combinations and recipe modifications, the information on fat could be derived from the fast method of Chapter Four. The difference is that when you construct such a table, you only need to list the figures in the column headed FAT. The PROT, CARBO, and CAL columns do not appear in your listing, and the calculations to produce the "% of calories" line are not needed. Only the information for the FOOD, AMT, and FAT columns are entered. The numbers in the fat column are then added up to give total grams of fat for comparison with your quota for one meal. Otherwise, the same modifications of mixtures and recipes and the same combinations of foods for each meal can be explored. Considering the importance of protein during pregnancy, a compromise would be to keep the PROT column, but skip the CARBO and CAL columns and the "% of calories" calculation. Simply add up the grams of protein and compare the result with the previously defined goal for protein intake.

Effects of Combining High and Low Fat Dishes

The surest way to develop a low fat meal is to use components that are each low in fat. Yet the advantage of the fat calculation method is that dishes which are high in fat by themselves may be useable in a meal that is otherwise low in fat. A favorite way to eat seafood is to dip it in melted butter, or preferably margarine to reduce saturated fats and cholesterol. Diet plans that achieve low fat by banning all high fat dishes would eliminate this gourmet dish from the menu. This may not be necessary, depending on how much margarine is used. For example, crab has a loose texture and soaks up a lot of margarine. Artificial crab legs have fish as the main ingredient and their more compressed texture holds less margarine.

To test the fat level of this combination, a measured amount of margarine could be melted in a small cup. Pieces of simulated crab leg would then be dipped into the cup and the residual margarine could be poured into a measuring device. Two ounces of such a prepared seafood product was found to absorb 1 1/2 teaspoons of margarine. This dipped seafood serving totaled 55% fat, which is almost double our maximum allowable fat level. However, consider its effect on a full meal:

FOOD	AMT	PROT	CARBO	FAT	CAL
Cherry yogurt	6 oz	7	32	4	190
Fish-crab legs	2 oz	7	4	0	47
Margarine	1 1/2 tsp	0	0	6	50
Corn kernels	1/3 cup	2	10	0	55
Bread, wheat	1 slice	3	14	1	65
Jelly	2 tsp	0	9	0	35
TOTALS		19	69	11	442
% by calories		17%	61%	22%	

This is a well balanced meal, supplying almost half the day's quota of protein for a non-pregnant woman, with carbohydrates providing the majority of calories and with the fat percentage falling at the bottom of the 20% to 30% range. The total of 11 grams of fat falls below the range of 15-22 grams for one meal. Even adding a dish of ice cream to this meal would only raise the total fat to 31%. However, the weight of fat would then be 25 grams, which is a little too high. Half a dish of ice cream would be a reasonable compromise. The extra work of making all these calculations is well worth the reward of having a wide choice of foods and being able to retain some favorite fatty foods in the diet.

Chapter Seven

THE MONTHS OF PREGNANCY

Assuming adjustments in dietary intake of fat have already been made, the state of pregnancy brings some special considerations. The best way to deal with these issues is to see a physician as early as possible, such as when pregnancy is being planned and before it actually occurs. The reason for getting advice early is that the critical period of pregnancy for avoiding birth defects is early. This can be understood by reviewing the events of conception and early development.

Development of the Embryo

The average time for discharge of an egg from the ovary and for fertilization is 14 days after the first day of the menstrual period. There is considerable individual variation around this average time. After the egg is fertilized, the egg cell divides into many cells that first form a ball. A few days later, fluid enters the ball of cells and blows it up into a tiny sphere, smaller than the head of a pin, called a blastocyst. This structure meanwhile has moved down the uterine tube and reached the uterus. A week after fertilization the blastocyst has attached to the inner wall of the uterus.

During the second week, cells inside the blastocyst form a flat disk, the beginning of an embryo. The earliest stage in the development of a nervous system appears during the third week. The third week is the time when the woman is expecting her next menstrual period. The placenta has released a hormone that prevents menstruation, so the woman usually suspects pregnancy for the first time at this stage of development. This third week of development is the start of the period in pregnancy when there is danger of birth defects. The woman should already be avoiding agents and conditions that carry a risk of causing birth defects.

Consult a Physician Early

One advantage of contacting a physician before getting pregnant is to anticipate and avoid problems at this early stage of embryonic development. Another advantage of counselling by a physician is to receive information specific to yourself. A physician who knows your medical history, work environment and other relevant aspects of your life can counsel you about your specific problems and risks. Thirdly, the physician is a source of current information, including the current status of anything written in this book. Due to the time required for publishing and distributing a book, it is usually written 9 months to a year before you buy it. Many new discoveries could be released at medical meetings or in medical journals during that time.

Birth Defects

The period of greatest risk for birth defects is during the fourth to ninth weeks of pregnancy. This is the time to be especially careful about exposure to drugs and other potentially toxic substances, also nutritional excesses or deficiencies. Large excesses or deficiencies of vitamins are potentially dangerous to the embryo, but minor variations should not cause a problem. Two common lifestyle habits that have an adverse effect are heavy intake of alcohol and smoking. Even moderate alcohol intake may not be safe, so the Surgeon General's report recommends that women avoid alcohol entirely during pregnancy.

The most thoroughly documented effect of smoking is an increased rate of late fetal and early neonatal death. That is, women who smoke during pregnancy, especially the final months, are more likely to have their baby die shortly before, or shortly after birth. The increased deaths among young babies of women smokers from such causes as respiratory problems and the sudden infant death syndrome may be due to passive exposure of the infant to smoke after birth. Smoking may also increase birth defects, but this is not as constant a finding as the perinatal death effect. Ideally, the embryo and fetus should be shielded from cigarette smoke throughout pregnancy and the newborn baby should be shielded from breathing sidestream smoke at least during the first few months after birth.

Drugs taken by the mother can be assumed to cross the placenta and affect the baby, unless there is clear evidence to the contrary. Furthermore, the effect of a drug on adults is not necessarily the effect it will have on the embryo. For example, the drug thalidomide had a sedative effect on the mother, but caused malformations of the limbs in the baby. Thousands of babies were affected before the cause was discovered. Despite 25 years of study since that tragedy happened, scientists still do not understand why thalidomide disrupted limb development. Obviously, drugs should not be taken during pregnancy for trivial reasons. Yet, a drug may be important for maternal health and a decision must be made by the physician as to whether this outweighs a possible risk to the embryo.

Some drugs are known to carry a small risk of producing birth defects, yet are used anyway because of their importance to the health of the woman who needs them. The hazard to the embryo from the mother's uncontrolled disease can be greater than the hazard of the drug. These risks need to be weighed by the physician, who will advise whether the drug should be continued or withdrawn.

The Fetal Period

The third month is the beginning of the fetal period. The general shape of almost all organs is well established by this time. An important phase of development in the early fetal period is the specialization of tissues. Several tissues make up an organ. Once the shape of the organ is established, the tissues start to develop their special functions. Cancer is a disease of tissues, not organs. Most cancers involve mainly one of the several tissues in an organ. Perhaps the reason the early fetal period seems to be the main time at which cancer is programmed prenatally relates to the fact that tissues are developing their special functions at this time. Regardless of theory, our best estimate so far is that dietary fat should be most carefully regulated during the third and fourth months of pregnancy.

Adequate Nutrition for Pregnancy

There are two broad nutritional issues for pregnancy. One is to assure sufficient food intake to cover the needs of both the mother and fetus. The second is to correct any nutritional deficiencies of the mother in advance of pregnancy. One illustration of the value of advance preparation concerns a birth defect of the nervous system. There is some evidence that starting the use of prenatal multivitamin pills one to three months before pregnancy lessens the chance of the baby being born with spina bifida and similar neural tube defects. Spina bifida is a condition where some vertebrae are incomplete and tissue, including the spinal cord, can protrude through the opening. The need for taking vitamins early is evident when the development of the vertebrae is considered. During the fourth week, the cells that will form the vertebrae are already surrounding the spinal cord. Remember that the fourth week of embryonic development comes just after the first missed menstrual period. If the woman waits until she is sure of pregnancy to correct a vitamin deficiency, she is starting too late to help the development of the embryo's vertebrae and spinal cord. The use of multivitamin pills in preparation for pregnancy should be limited to pills with vitamin content not exceeding recommended daily allowances, unless prescribed by a physician.

Another reason for developing good nutritional habits before pregnancy concerns evidence that the fetus can draw on maternal stores of nutrients. If the mother has a good store of vitamins and minerals at the start of pregnancy, this is some assurance that minor deficiencies in diet during pregnancy can be compensated. An important lesson was learned from the period of food shortage in Holland near the end of the second world war. Near starvation conditions prevailed for a few months. Yet, the effects on children born during that time were minimal. This was attributed to the women being in a good nutritional state before pregnancy The opposite condition can be found in certain developing countries where some people are chronically malnourished. When malnourished women become pregnant, an adverse effect of this condition on the fetus can be recognized.

Recommended Intake of Nutrients

The government has issued a set of recommended daily dietary allowances for infants, children, men and women, including pregnant and lactating women. I have listed the figures for adult women of childbearing age in the table on the next page. The figures for mature, non-pregnant women are listed first in the table. This is to encourage you to strive for good nutrition at the non-pregnant level before pregnancy starts. The second column of figures lists the extra amounts necessary during pregnancy. The third column just summates the first two columns to give the total amount of each nutrient needed during pregnancy.

There are reasons why a woman need not be excessively compulsive about meeting these recommendations exactly. One reason is that they are estimates, and some authorities have arrived at slightly different estimates. Secondly, as already mentioned, the fetus probably can draw from the mother's stores of vitamins and minerals, and so is not entirely dependent on day to day dietary intake of the mother.

NUTRIENT	BEFORE PREGNANCY	PREGNANCY SUPPLEMENT	PREGNANCY TOTAL
Protein	44 g	30 g	74 g
Vitamin A	800 µg	200 µg	1000 µg
Vitamin D	7.5 µg	5 µg	12.5 µg
Vitamin E	8 mg	2 mg	10 mg
Vitamin C	60 mg	20 mg	80 mg
Thiamin	1.1 mg	0.4 mg	1.5 mg
Riboflavin	1.3 mg	0.3 mg	1.6 mg
Niacin	14 mg	2 mg	16 mg
Vitamin B-6	2 mg	0.6 mg	2.6 mg
Folacin	400 µg	400 µg	800 µg
Vitamin B-12	3 µg	1 µg	4 µg
Calcium	800 mg	400 mg	1200 mg
Phosphorus	800 mg	400 mg	1200 mg
Magnesium	300 mg	150 mg	450 mg
Iron	18 mg	*	*
Zinc	15 mg	5 mg	20 mg
Iodine	150 µg	25 µg	175 µg

*   An asterisk is used in the last two columns for iron because the table on recommended daily allowances did not list an additional amount of iron from diet. Instead, a supplemental pill with 30-60 mg of iron was suggested.

Physician Guidance for Nutrients

Faced with this complicated array of nutrient requirements, the physician will usually resort to one of three options:
(1) Depend on the adequacy of the patient's diet to meet all of these recommended dietary intakes.

(2)   Supplement selectively, for example with iron and folacin.

(3)   Use a complete vitamin and mineral supplement.

     The patient's dietary history is useful in arriving at a decision.   If you have written out some tables like those recommended in previous chapters, they should be helpful. For example, the protein totals will show whether protein intake is adequate.   The physician may be concerned about total caloric intake.   If calories are included in the percent fat tables, as shown in the previous chapters, this information could be useful to the physician also.   One authority has recommended a daily increase of 300 calories during pregnancy. Another has recommended a minimum total intake per day of 2000 calories.   However, total calories needed depends on the individual's level of exercise and metabolic activity.   The physician may depend on rate of weight gain during pregnancy to advise on caloric intake.

     Some people regularly consume vitamin pills. Women of childbearing age who use such pills should be sure they do not contain multiples of the recommended allowances in the preceding table unless prescribed by a physician.   The reason is that some nutrients may be toxic to the fetus if taken in excess.   Large doses of vitamin A can cause birth defects in laboratory animals.   With the possible exception of unusual foods like fish liver, it is considered unlikely that a dangerous excess of vitamins would come from foods.   The main concern is with pills containing excessive doses above those recommended for the average person.

Compromises

Ideally, everyone would keep fat in the range of 20% to 30% for all meals and snacks at home, at parties and in restaurants and consume other nutrients close to the levels specified in the table of recommended daily allowances. Few, if any people will reach this level of diet control. Therefore, it is important to recognize several levels of accomplishment. First priority for fat is to avoid meals loaded with fatty foods during pregnancy, and probably especially during the second through fourth months. This can be accomplished to a considerable extent by reviewing the table on fat content of foods at the end of this book. Such a minimal effort is better than doing nothing and might have some impact on the cancer problem. The next level is to analyze typical recipes and meals and make adjustments to avoid repetitive indulgence in high fat meals. The final practical level is to have most meals in the 20% to 30% fat range and avoid any meals that are exceptionally high in fat. This is a reasonable compromise. If combined with stricter control during the first half of pregnancy, it should be sufficient to protect the fetus.

Caution

The preceding paragraph concedes that a weak effort to control fat intake during pregnancy is probably better than no effort at all. This does not mean that the sensitive period for fat exposure is definitely, or exclusively during pregnancy. Human studies on cancer and nutrition only cite "early in life" and not pregnancy specifically. My experiment with mice utilized fat-controlled diets from sexual maturity, through pregnancy, to delivery of the pups. Citing the first half of pregnancy as the sensitive period is only a current "best guess." Every effort should be made to control dietary fat intake throughout the reproductive years.

Chapter Eight

WEIGHT CONTROL BEFORE PREGNANCY

The words "before pregnancy" are in the title of this chapter to emphasize that a vigorous weight loss program should not be attempted during pregnancy. It could deprive the fetus of nutrients and energy. Of course, almost everyone knows this anyway. Weight control during pregnancy should be directed only at the amount of weight gain reasonably allowed for growth of the uterus, placenta and fetus. Your physician can be expected to provide counselling on this matter.

Obesity is well recognized as being dangerous to your health. For example, it is an independent risk factor for heart attack. Innumerable books have been written on weight loss dieting. So why bring this subject up in a book about pregnancy? There are two reasons. The first concerns cancer and the fetus.

Obesity and Cancer

Is there any evidence linking obesity with cancer? Studies of women with uterine cancer have repeatedly and consistently linked this disease with obesity. Looking for a reason to explain this link has led to evidence that obesity upsets hormone balance by increasing the amount of estrogen in the body. Since DES, which is a synthetic estrogen, programs the fetus for cancer, it is reasonable to question whether excess estrogen from obesity could do the same.

Hormone balance during pregnancy is very different from hormone balance during the postmenopausal period when uterine cancer is most likely to occur. Some scientists believe the levels of estrogen are so high during pregnancy that any effect of obesity on estrogen levels would be too small to have an effect. However, the obesity may change the amount of a protein in the blood that binds estrogen and change the amount of estrogen free in the blood stream. Theoretical arguments do not settle such issues. Performing experiments and collecting evidence is the only solution.

Cancer in Male Offspring

Is there any evidence that obesity can program the human fetus for cancer? A link between maternal body weight and testicular cancer of sons was described in Chapter Two. A similar study was performed in relation to undescended testes in newborn babies. Again obesity of the mother was a risk factor. The relevance of undescended testes to cancer is that babies born with undescended testes are at higher risk of developing testicular cancer later in life.

Does this mean that maternal obesity programs the fetus for cancer? Such a direct cause-and-effect conclusion cannot be drawn from this type of risk factor study. The reason is that excess maternal weight may just be a marker for some other condition that is more likely to be present in obese women than in non-obese women. The usual way to test for causation is to run an experiment in which other factors are controlled and only the obesity factor changes. This is difficult to do in human studies. It is usually done with animal experimentation after human studies show that the problem is worth exploring.

Cancer and Calories

Another line of reasoning comes from attempts to explain the international differences in cancer rates that seem to depend on dietary differences. When no consistent relation was found within a country between adult intake of fat and rate of breast cancer, scientists questioned whether the real factor was excess calories rather than excess fat in the diet. The reasons for this suspicion are first in relation to food energy. Fat has over twice as many calories as protein and carbohydrate, specifically, 9 calories per gram of fat compared to 4 calories per gram for the other two nutrients. Secondly, sugar intake tends to parallel fat intake between countries and both sugary and fatty foods taste exceptionally good and will tend to promote overeating. Finally, sugar and fat tend to occur in foods low in fiber and bulk, which can affect appetite. The net result of all three factors is excess calories. Excess calories cause obesity. Therefore, the large international differences in cancer rate may be due to obesity, with dietary fat being only one factor. Since the international differences seem to be operating early in life for reproductive system cancer, obesity may be acting during pregnancy. Again, a direct test of this issue needs to come from animal experimentation.

Testing for an Obesity Factor

Do animal studies prove that obesity programs the fetus for cancer? Surprisingly, no such animal experiments have been published. In the experiment I performed with varied amounts of fat in the diet, all the pregnant mice were young and not obese. They were one to two months old and lean, weighing between 20 and 30 grams. Therefore, this experiment demonstrated an effect of dietary fat independent of any possible obesity factor.

As mice of this strain grow older, they tend to grow fat. By four months of age they average 40 grams and by 8 months about 50 grams. I have some preliminary evidence that the cancer rate in the offspring rises with rising maternal age. Therefore, this increased cancer rate may be due to maternal obesity. However, the offspring were

"DES granddaughter" mice, and other changes with maternal age may have been occurring. The issue could be tested by comparing mice allowed to eat all they want, and thus become obese, with mice on a food-restricted diet to prevent obesity. I intend to do this if I can raise the necessary funds.

In summary, if you are already pregnant and obese, do not worry. There is not enough evidence linking obesity during pregnancy with cancer to consider this a serious issue yet. On the other hand, if you are obese and not pregnant, the possibility of an effect during pregnancy is just one more reason for attempting weight control.

Weight Control

The second reason for raising the issue of weight control in this book is that controlling fat intake provides an excellent opportunity to control weight. For the reasons cited above, a low fat diet is less likely to cause a weight increase than a high fat diet. Nevertheless, the final outcome depends on the balance between caloric intake and caloric expenditure. Most people who eat more calories than they burn will put on fat. If you analyze your meals by constructing the type of table explained in the previous chapters, it will be easy to see which of the foods you eat are contributing the most calories to your diet. It is essential to include snacks in these calculations, both to keep track of fat and to keep track of calories.

Low Fat vs. Low Calories

A low fat meal is not necessarily a low calorie meal. In Chapter Six, adding half a dish of ice cream to the crab leg meal did not raise the fat level above the restricted level. However, see what it did to the caloric content of the meal! The next table shows the meal without, and with a half a dish of ice cream.

FOOD	AMT	PROT	CARBO	FAT	CAL
Cherry yogurt	6 oz	7	32	4	190
Fish-crab legs	2 oz	7	4	0	47
Margarine	1 1/2 tsp	0	0	6	50
Corn kernels	1/3 cup	2	10	0	55
Bread, wheat	1 slice	3	14	1	65
Jelly	2 tsp	0	9	0	35
TOTALS		19	69	11	442
Ice cream	1/2 cup	3	16	7	135
NEW TOTALS		22	85	18	577

The fat content is 27%, which is near the middle of the percentage range. Similarly, the 18 grams is in the middle of the 15 to 22 gram range. However, adding the half dish of ice cream increased the total calories for the meal from 442 to 577. This is a 31% increase. The meal still has an acceptable fat level, but now the caloric content is much higher than it was without the ice cream. Can you afford the extra calories?

Cumulative Caloric Intake

A single day provides a convenient time span for planning caloric intake. For example, the last breakfast listed in Chapter Five could be combined with the revised crab leg luncheon on the previous page and the turkey tetrazini dinner in Chapter Six. Using only totals from these meals the result can be seen in the next table.

FOOD	AMT	PROT	CARBO	FAT	CAL
Breakfast	1	20	68	12	448
Lunch	1	22	85	18	577
Dinner	1	50	97	16	730
TOTALS	3 meals	92	250	46	1755

With these three meals, the intake of protein is 92 grams which moderately exceeds the 74 grams recommended for pregnancy. The percent fat is 23%, predictably within the specified range, since each meal was low fat. Similarly, the total fat for the day was 46 grams, which approximates the lower limit of the 44-67 gram daily intake range for an average woman. The total calories for the day would be 1755, assuming there were no snacks to be added. Is this about right, too many, or too few? It depends on the calories specified for someone of your age, sex, height, and level of activity, as described in Chapter Four. It also depends on whether you are trying to hold your present weight, lose weight, or gain weight. It would be low for pregnancy, where weight gain is needed and a minimum of 2000 calories has been suggested. In contrast, it might be appropriate for a non-pregnant, slightly overweight person.

Setting an Ideal Weight

What is your ideal weight? Tables of average weight for a given height provide a starting point. They can give a somewhat better estimate if they allow for bone size, for example by utilizing wrist measurements as a clue to bone thickness. However, they do not allow for differences in amount of muscle compared to fat. The most reliable method involves computing the percent fat in the body. Considerable accuracy can be attained by measurements involving submersion in a tank of water. Such a complicated system is accessible to very few people. Fortunately, another method almost as accurate is easily accessible. It only requires use of a pair of skinfold thickness calipers.

The technique of measuring the thickness of a fold of skin is very simple. A pinch of skin on a specific part of the body is measured by an instrument that works like a pair of pliers. It has a scale that shows how far open it is being held by the fold of skin. A booklet that comes with the instrument has pictures showing where to take the measurements, as well as tables that list the percent body fat represented by the measurement. The method is definitely as accurate as anyone needs for deciding on an ideal weight. Physicians may use expensive metal calipers, but plastic calipers are adequate for the average person. They

can be shared with family and friends, because
they are not needed on a daily basis. The
accompanying booklet will give recommended
ranges of percent body fat that are reasonably
conservative. If skinfold calipers are not
available locally, they can be purchased by mail
order. One source is Creative Health Products,
5148 Saddle Ridge Road, Plymouth, Michigan,
48170; by telephone, area 313, 453-5309. Exercise
is an important component of a moderate weight
loss program to assure that muscle mass is retained
while fat is being converted to energy. If a person
exercises while dieting, muscle will get food
components preferentially, while fat gets burned
off. This works well down to a reasonable level of
body fat, like 16% for men and 20% for women.
Very low ranges achieved by athletes, such as 10%
for men and 15% for women, are not recommended
for the average person. One reason is that the
very low levels are best reached by intensive
exercise, not intensive dieting. The potential
danger of excessive dieting is that non-fat tissue
will tend to be lost as well as fat, even with a
moderately brisk exercise program. This is not a
problem with reasonable objectives like 14% to
18% for men and 18% to 24% for women. Another
reason for women is that it may interfere with
fertility.

Fertility and Body Fat

The Surgeon General's report recommended
that prepregnant weight not go below 85% of

standard weight for height. Unfortunately, this statement is of limited value in relation to percent body fat, since standard weight tables may not deal with bone size and would not allow for muscle development. Some figures have been published for percent body fat in relation to fertility; for example, a minimum of 17% body fat for menarche and 22% for maintenance of female reproductive ability.

The possibility has been raised that higher levels like 26% to 28% may favor ability to reproduce. Yet, lower levels of fat correlate with less risk of reproductive system cancer. These conflicting goals have led to speculation that lower body fat levels during the teenage period and more normal levels during optimal reproductive years might be a good compromise. Thus, a woman planning to become pregnant might reasonably chose a 22% to 28% target range for total body fat. This still represents a trim body shape. For many women, reaching 22% to 28% would mean limiting amount of weight loss rather than adding weight. However, if weight needs to be added, be sure to do this with extra calories from complex carbohydrates and not by increasing fat intake above the level recommended for amount of calories in the diet. Of course, increasing calories to add body fat would increase the allowance of dietary fat per day. The issue is to not exceed 20% to 30% of calories from fat. In other words, if food intake is increased to gain weight, keep the increase in fat proportionate to the increase in calories. The body can build fat from any calories, it does not need fatty foods to build body fat.

A Comprehensive Weight Loss Program

A sensible weight loss program has several elements. The first step is to decide on an ideal weight by weight tables, or preferably by skinfold calipers. Assuming the ideal weight is lower than your present weight, the next step is to develop a fat-controlled diet, as explained in the previous chapters. This type of diet will help with weight control by limiting intake of "fattening" foods and also provide a starting point for calorie control. Stay on the new diet a few weeks and weigh yourself daily. If your weight is holding constant or rising, then evaluate your level of physical activity.

Everyone needs to engage in a type of activity that will benefit their cardiovascular system, that is, a type of exercise that will help prevent heart attack. A standard recommendation by exercise physiologists is to exercise three times a week for 30 minutes at each session. The exercise should be sufficiently vigorous to raise heart rate and usually to cause sweating. Books on aerobic exercise usually provide information on how to calculate an appropriate heart rate range. A person with any symptoms of disease, or significantly overweight, should check with a physician before starting an exercise program. Age is also a factor. The older a person is before starting exercise, the more important it becomes to be cleared for exercise by a physician. The American Heart Association has a booklet explaining how to start an exercise program and listing the various physical conditions which signal the need to see a physician before starting to exercise. Many books on aerobic exercise carry similar warnings.

Aerobic Exercises

Good aerobic exercises are jogging, bicycling, swimming, canoeing, rowing, cross-country skiing, fast walking and other activities that maintain a steady vigorous pace of exercise. Indoor aerobic exercises include stationary bicycles, rowing machines and cross-country ski machines. Aerobic dance classes can be followed up at home with records or VCR tapes. The most important steps are to find activities you like and to continue exercising throughout the year. Start an exercise program gradually, with limited intensity and duration. Exercise is such an important part of staying healthy that it should be a given high priority. Buy a good, authoritative book on exercising and pick a program designed for your age and fitness level.

Regulating Food Intake

Assuming a good aerobic exercise program is being carried out on a regular basis, we can return to the issue of diet and weight reduction. If you are losing one or two pounds every week or two, just maintain the same caloric intake until optimal weight is reached, then add a few extra calories to hold at that weight. If your weight is not decreasing, remove some food items from the diet, or reduce the size of some servings. Continue daily weighing and hold the menu constant when weight starts to decrease at the rate of a pound or two every one to two weeks. Extreme obesity, or medical problems related to weight may require a more vigorous weight reduction program under medical supervision.

There are two advantages to this method of weight loss compared to special diets only used for a limited period. One is that the diet should be nutritionally satisfactory, since the food changes needed for weight loss are minor. Secondly, the change back to a standard diet adds only a few more calories and can be tailored to hold weight steady. A major problem with obesity and dieting is that a large proportion of dieters who lose weight regain it again, presumably by returning to poor eating habits.

Chapter Nine

FAMILY MEALS

Meals that are shared provide a wonderful opportunity for health benefits to be shared - which means sharing the work, too. There is no reason why the cook should do all the percent fat and calorie calculations, unless that person enjoys the task. A fat-controlled diet for pregnancy forms an ideal base for a healthy diet to benefit everyone. This fact will become obvious when the principles of a healthy diet are reviewed.

Years ago, a good diet meant one with enough protein, vitamins and minerals. This is still true as a starting point. The broad approach to including these nutrients is to build a diet with a variety of fresh foods covering the main categories of meat, fish, grains, fruits and vegetables. However, some specific inclusions and exclusions have arisen on the basis of studying dietary risk factors of the major diseases.

Diet and Diseases

According to the Surgeon General's report, the total number of deaths in this country are divided among the ten major causes as follows: heart disease 35.7%, cancer 22.4%, cerebrovascular disease (stroke) 7%, accidents 4.4%, chronic obstructive lung disease 3.7%, pneumonia and influenza 3.2%, diabetes mellitus 1.8%, suicide 1.4%, cirrhosis of the liver 1.2%, arteriosclerosis 1.1%. Eight of these are related to lifestyle. Tobacco has a major role in causing heart disease and cancer. Alcohol is involved in accidents, suicide, cancer and liver cirrhosis. Diet is a significant factor in heart disease, stroke, cancer, diabetes and atherosclerosis. Altogether, lifestyle was involved in almost 1.5 million of the 2.1 million total deaths in 1987. This makes it exceptionally worthwhile to spend some time designing family meals and becoming used to new eating habits.

The Surgeon General's report makes the following recommendations:
1. Eat a variety of foods.
2. Maintain desirable weight.
3. Avoid too much fat, saturated fat, and cholesterol.
4. Eat foods with adequate starch and fiber.
5. Avoid too much sugar.
6. Avoid too much sodium.
7. If you drink alcoholic beverages, do so in moderation.

The report expands on these recommendations with detailed comments directed to the average person, as follows:

Fats and cholesterol: Reduce consumption of fat (especially saturated fat) and cholesterol. Choose foods relatively low in these substances, such as vegetables, fruits, whole grain foods, fish, poultry, lean meats, and low-fat dairy products. Use food preparation methods that add little or no fat.

Energy and weight control: Achieve and maintain a desirable body weight. To do so, choose a dietary pattern in which energy (caloric) intake is consistent with energy expenditure. To reduce energy intake, limit consumption of foods relatively high in calories, fats, and sugars, and minimize alcohol consumption. Increase energy expenditure through regular and sustained physical activity.

Complex carbohydrates and fiber: Increase consumption of whole grain foods and cereal products, vegetables (including dried beans and peas), and fruits.

Sodium: Reduce intake of sodium by choosing foods relatively low in sodium and limiting the amount of salt added in food preparation and at the table.

Alcohol: To reduce the risk for chronic disease, take alcohol only in moderation (no more than two drinks a day), if at all. Avoid drinking any alcohol before or while driving, operating machinery, taking medications, or engaging in any other activity requiring judgement. Avoid drinking alcohol while pregnant.

The report has additional recommendations for some people:

Fluoride: Community water systems should contain fluoride at optimal levels for prevention of tooth decay. If such water is not available, use other appropriate sources of fluoride.

Sugars: Those who are particularly vulnerable to dental caries (cavities), especially children, should limit their consumption and frequency of use of foods high in sugars.

Calcium: Adolescent girls and adult women should increase consumption of foods high in calcium, including low-fat dairy products.

Iron: Children, adolescents, and women of childbearing age should be sure to consume foods that are good sources of iron, such as lean meats, fish, certain beans, and iron-enriched cereals and whole grain products. The issue is of special concern for low-income families.

Also, the report has a section devoted to maternal and child nutrition. The 78 page booklet is entitled "Summary and Recommendations. The Surgeon General's Report on Nutrition and Health." This booklet is available for $2.75. To order the booklet, request it by the above title and send a check to:

Superintendent of Documents
Government Printing Office
Washington, D.C. 20402-9325

Disease and Dietary Fat

An encouraging fact is that if you have followed the recommendations in this book so far, then the major part of the job has already been done. The American Heart Association, the National Cancer Institute, the American Cancer Society and the Surgeon General all agree that the amount of fat in the diet should be reduced to 30% of calories, or less. The approximate minimum of 20% that I have been recommending is directed only towards pregnancy. For people whose concern is heart attack and other fat-related diseases, this minimum of 20% does not necessarily apply. Someone with sufficiently high cholesterol levels to require stringent control measures should be under a physician's supervision and receive dietary advice specific to their problem.

Types of Fat

Several qualifications can be made in the fat story. Some fats are considered worse than others. If you are going to start reducing fats, you might as well get rid of the worst ones first. Saturated fats are considered the most dangerous for heart disease. Animal fats are typically high in saturated fats. Animal fats also show the strongest correlation with cancer, internationally. Obviously, the first place to reduce fat in the diet is with animal fats. Scanning the food tables at the back of this book will quickly reveal the main culprits. For example, reading down from the first page, bacon is 82% fat, rib roast is 81% fat, bologna is 86% fat, and so on. If it is not practical to eliminate these foods from the diet, the alternative is to serve them infrequently and to use small portions. Some vegetable oils are high in saturated fats too, like palm oil and coconut oil, and substantial intake of these oils should be avoided.

The problem of cholesterol is partly solved by the fact that the high cholesterol foods are animal foods. Most of these need to be reduced anyway, because of their high content of saturated fats. Foods high in cholesterol are eggs, meat, poultry, seafood, and dairy products. Yet, poultry and seafood are not as high in total fat as most other meats, so are preferable. A similar qualification can be made for low-fat dairy products. Eggs and organ meats like liver are especially high in cholesterol. In contrast, fruits, vegetables, grains and nuts are free of cholesterol. However, nuts are very high in fat, so must always be included with calculations of a fat-controlled meal.

The other qualification in the fat story pertains to fish fat. The omega-3 polyunsaturated acids in fish have been shown to help in prevention of heart attack. Fish that are rich in these particular compounds are salmon, mackeral, herring, tuna, bluefish, whiting, trout, and some lesser known species. However, many other fish also have some polyunsaturated fatty acids. Effects of fish fat on the human fetus are not known. Since a number of cultures have a diet rich in fish, including the Japanese, presumably fish are a reasonable part of the diet during pregnancy. However, extreme measures like taking fish oil capsules should be avoided until there has been time for more research.

Salt

Another main issue for a diet designed to protect the heart is sodium. Food labels list sodium in milligrams (mg). The National Research Council recommends 1100 to 3300 mg. of sodium per day. The problem is not in getting enough sodium. The problem is in getting too much sodium. The average American consumes 4000 to 6000 mg. of sodium every day. Sodium intake should be reduced to the recommended range. Opinions about salt intake during pregnancy have tended to vary, so consult your physician on this issue. One way to become aware of your salt consumption is to read the food labels. Some foods, like potato chips, may not list the amount of salt, but the hazard is self evident. Many foods that are modified before packaging are high in sodium, like cured meats, many canned goods and commercially prepared main courses. A logical precaution is to be aware of major sources of sodium in your diet and minimize intake of the highly salted items.

Some highly salted foods are pickles, olives, salted nuts, soy sauce, hot dogs, bacon, processed cheese, canned soups, various snack chips, salted pretzels, canned fish, luncheon meats, ham, catsup, and canned meats.

Salt may be a factor in cancer, too. Intake of salt-cured, smoked and nitrite-cured foods should be limited. Since meats prepared in this manner are also typically high in fat, a good policy is to eliminate them entirely from the diet, especially during pregnancy. Nitrosamines are formed in the stomach from nitrites. Nitrosamines given to pregnant animals are very potent for inducing brain tumors in the offspring. Eating habits were compared between mothers whose children developed brain tumors and mothers of children without brain tumors. The mothers of the brain tumor children had eaten more nitrite-preserved foods.

Diet Books for Cardiovascular Disease

If someone in the family is already using a special diet book for prevention of heart attack, this book might serve as an additional source of basic dietary information. The book may contain tables of food values that could supplement those at the end of this book. Such tables would probably contain information on types of fat and on cholesterol content. Listings of cholesterol content per meal could be added to the tables developed previously in Chapters Five and Six. The objective would be to avoid daily intake of cholesterol in excess of 250 to 300 mg. Such books may also carry low fat recipes with the protein, carbohydrate and fat content specified. These recipes could be useful in building low fat meals, as explained in previous chapters.

The full text of the Surgeon General's report recommended that all Americans, except children under age 2, derive less than 10% of calories from saturated fats. This was accompanied by a warning to make sure children receive an adequate intake of total calories. The additional calories could come from complex carbohydrates. Fat restriction for children should not be so vigorous as to interfere with adequate nutrition.

Tracking all types of fat, in addition to the other calculations recommended specifically for pregnancy, would add up to considerable work. Whether this is justified would depend on the family's level of concern for cardiovascular disease. Listing cholesterol is probably the easiest addition to make. A reasonable priority sequence would be to control total dietary fat first, then proceed to check cholesterol content. Finally, an awareness of the sources of saturated fats would add additional sophistication to food choices. However, if the family is at special risk due to genetic background, or medical history, a more intensive effort might be needed.

Anti-cancer Foods

Tired of being asked to eliminate foods? The good news is that some foods probably help to prevent cancer. High fiber may help prevent colon cancer. Since fiber content tends to be low in fatty foods and high in grains, vegetables and fruits, the fat-controlled diet will tend to increase fiber intake. Including a high fiber cereal at breakfast provides further assurance. Cruciferous vegetables like cabbage, broccoli, Brussels sprouts, kohlrabi and cauliflower are also believed to help prevent cancer of the digestive tract.

People whose diet is rich in foods containing vitamin A and vitamin C tend to have a reduced cancer rate. Since factors other than the vitamins may be involved, intake of vitamin pills is not necessarily equivalent for cancer protection. Therefore, foods rich in these vitamins have been listed at the end of this book. The second set of tables lists foods with a useful amount of vitamin A. The third table lists food sources for vitamin C. Vitamin content has been expressed in terms of percent of the recommended daily allowance. Again, it is worth mentioning that excessive amounts of vitamin A are probably toxic to the fetus, based on animal studies. Toxic doses are not expected to arise from food, but could be delivered by mega-dose vitamin pills.

Diet and Lifespan

The profile of a person with high odds of premature aging and early onset of fatal illness is well known to medical science. This person is a heavy drinker and smoker, overindulges in foods high in fat and sugar, has a sedentary lifestyle, is overweight, and does little to counterbalance stress.

The powerful effect that just diet alone can have on lifespan was demonstrated long ago with animal experiments. Mice kept on a calorie restricted diet averaged a longer lifespan than mice allowed to eat all they wanted. Equally important, onset of diseases like cancer were postponed. When the diet was low in fat, the effects on cancer prevention were even more pronounced.

Changing diet and lifestyle takes time. How much time do you have? Not much today, of course. But what about in your lifetime? How soon can you afford to start feeling sickly, to become terminally ill? Have you saved some dreams for the future? Save some healthy years, too.

Chapter Ten

"ASK YOUR MOTHER"

Were you born anytime during the period of the 1940's to the early 1970's? If so, you may have been exposed to DES before birth. "Ask your mother." This is a slogan of the DES Action organization - a group of DES daughters, sons and mothers who have been trying to help people in respect to the DES problem. The first step is helping people find out whether they have been exposed. This is not as easy as it may seem. If your mother remembers taking the drug and the hospital or physician's records confirm that it was DES, then you can be reasonably sure of exposure. However, ruling out exposure is much more difficult. A large group of mothers who had taken DES during pregnancy were identified by hospital records. They were sent a questionnaire asking them what drugs they had taken during pregnancy. Many remembered taking DES, but 29% did not remember and 8% claimed they definitely had not taken DES even though the hospital records contradicted this claim. As would be expected, about one third of DES daughters do not know they are DES daughters.

Importance of DES Exposure

Why is it important for someone to know whether they were exposed prenatally to DES? One strong reason is to be aware of a special cancer risk and to seek appropriate medical care. The risk is for a rare glandular form of vaginal and cervical cancer. Fortunately, the risk of a DES daughter developing this cancer at a young age is only one in a thousand. This risk may seem too low to justify repeated medical examinations. Yet, the examinations can be done at the same time as screening for the common type of cervical cancer. Furthermore, there is mounting evidence that DES daughters are more susceptible to the common form of cervical cancer. Thus, regular gynecologic exams are especially important for DES daughters. Some of the screening steps for DES-related cancer are not part of a routine checkup, so it is important to let the physician know if you have been exposed to DES.

Current Information on DES

About 10 years ago, some DES mothers and daughters developed an organization to help each other and to lobby for progress in solving the DES problem. They currently issue a news letter to keep their membership informed on medical, legal, and legislative developments in regard to DES. There are affiliated groups in most states and in several other countries where members meet to exchange concerns and work for the cause. The west coast office address is: DES Action, 2845 24th Street, San Francisco, CA 94110. The east coast office address is: DES Action, L.I. Jewish Medical Center, New Hyde Park, N.Y., 11040.

DES Exposure and Pregnancy Diet

My reason for raising the issue of DES exposure relates directly to the subject of this book - programming the fetus for cancer through high levels of dietary fat. The fetus of a DES daughter may be even more susceptible to cancer programming by dietary fat than the fetus of a non-exposed woman. The explanation begins with some research I performed several years ago. I injected some pregnant mice with DES, raised their female offspring, let the latter get pregnant, then raised their female offspring. These third generation female mice had a lot of reproductive tract cancer, even though they had never been directly exposed to DES.

The press reported this study, pointing out that the DES cancer risk may not stop with DES daughters, but may be passed on to "DES granddaughters." Physicians were quick to say that this was only a mouse experiment and may not apply to people. Yet, most cancer is linked to aging. If we wait until the third generation question is settled for the human population it will probably be much too late to apply preventive measures during pregnancy. Is it possible to reduce the transmission of a DES cancer risk to the fetus? The answer for mice is clearly yes. As reported in Chapter Two, the higher the dietary fat, the greater the incidence of cancer in DES granddaughter mice. The latter were used on the assumption that they would serve as a sensitive probe for a cancer increase from fat. They were not used for the purpose of finding a way to prevent the DES granddaughter effect. Nevertheless the experiment can be reinterpreted for that purpose.

Preventing the DES Granddaughter Effect

When the amount of fat in the diet of DES daughter mice was increased, the amount of cancer in the DES granddaughter mice increased. However, the highest levels of fat, namely, 36% and 49%, are equivalent to the average and upper range of fat content in the American diet. Therefore, reducing dietary fat should reduce the transmission of a DES cancer risk to granddaughters. DES daughters have a chance to protect their offspring by reducing the amount of fat they consume when they are pregnant. However, whereas the link between dietary fat during pregnancy and cancer in the offspring is based on both human and animal data for the general population, the connection is based only on animal data for the DES granddaughter effect. Therefore, consideration of possible mechanisms is justified. If a combined effect of DES and dietary fat makes sense biologically, then we can have more confidence that the mouse data are relevant to people.

Cancer from DES and Dietary Fat

A number of cancer-producing chemicals have been shown to produce a continuing cancer risk from generation to generation in laboratory animals, even though the chemical itself quickly disappears. The mechanism for this continued effect is not known, except in cases where the germ cells (sperm or egg) are known to have been mutated. Therefore, germ cell mutation is a possibility for DES. Another possibility is a repeating effect on prenatal development of the hypothalamus. In Chapter Two an explanation was provided for a possible link between abnormal development of the hypothalamus and a predisposition to cancer later in life. This same explanation can be used for the granddaughter effect. If an abnormal hypothalamus can upset hormone balance enough to predispose to cancer, it could also upset the hormones that reach the fetus from the mother and upset the development of the fetal hypothalamus. Thus, the third generation would also have abnormal hormones and an increased risk for cancer.

Explaining how dietary fat could fit into this picture requires a more detailed explanation of how DES causes cancer. Actually, this issue is not settled. Only one of several postulated mechanisms seems to relate to fat. This mechanism concerns the control of differentiation of the hypothalamus. Apparently the natural female hormone estrogen controls the differentiation of the hypothalamus. The fetus receives estrogen from the mother and it is also made by the placenta. So there is a lot of estrogen in the fetus, but most of it does not get into the hypothalamus. The reason is that most of the estrogen is firmly attached to a protein in the fetal blood called alpha-fetoprotein (AFP). AFP enters some parts of the brain, but not the hypothalamus. Thus, very little estrogen gets into the hypothalamus. If something goes wrong and a lot of estrogen enters the hypothalamus, this upsets its development and the fetus will grow up to have an abnormal hormone balance.

DES and the Hypothalamus

DES increases the size of a part of the hypothalamus that can be used as a marker for an estrogenic effect in rats. This means that DES probably altered hypothalamic differentiation. There are two ways it might be doing this. DES is not well bound to AFP, so it is free to enter the hypothalamus, where it may act in a manner similar to natural estrogen. The other possibility relates to evidence that DES can displace some natural estrogen from AFP and this extra free estrogen would then be able to enter the hypothalamus. This possibility is interesting in relation to fat. When dietary fat is digested, fatty acids are produced. Fatty acids also attach to AFP and can displace estrogen from the AFP, thus increasing the amount of free estrogen in the blood. If this happened in the fetal blood at the time the hypothalamus was differentiating, it could be expected to upset the development of the fetal hypothalamus and lead to increased risk of cancer later in life. This may be the explanation for the increased number of pituitary and uterine tumors seen in the offspring of pregnant mice on a high fat diet. Thus, DES and fat may both act by upsetting hypothalamic development. If the DES granddaughter effect is due to a perpetuation of the abnormal hypothalamus condition, as explained above, then the fatty diet could be aggravating this condition and producing the exceptionally high tumor rate seen in the mouse experiment. Remember that the DES tumor effect in people is well established. Secondly, the tumor effect of high fat diet in people is well supported by epidemiologic studies. The theoretical explanation for associating these two effects should be persuasive, even without the mouse experiment. Therefore, all DES daughters should make an intensive effort to avoid a high fat diet during pregnancy.

The Need for DES Research

A low fat diet during DES daughter pregnancies has great potential for minimizing the chance of cancer risk transmission to DES granddaughters. Unfortunately, a great many DES granddaughters were born before this preventive measure was discovered. Therefore, some new strategy is needed to protect those already born. You could protest that the third generation effect has not been proven for the human species, so all this worry and work could be for nothing. So we need more evidence to decide whether there really is a cancer risk for the third generation. This needs to be done without waiting to see if granddaughters develop DES-related cancer, so that preventive measures can be developed soon enough to be effective. We need to discover what changes take place early in life that predispose to cancer later in life. If these changes are discovered in the mouse, then evidence for similar changes can be looked for in DES granddaughters. This should establish whether the latter really are at risk for DES-related cancer.

Mechanism of Third Generation Cancer Transmission

At least two mechanisms can be suggested to explain the transmission of an increased cancer risk to the third generation. One possibility is that DES mutated the egg cells of the DES daughter when she was a fetus. Incidentally, if this is true, then DES sons should be at equal risk of passing on a DES cancer risk to their children, since presumably their sperm cells would also be mutated. The second possibility involves differentiation of the hypothalamus, as mentioned before. If DES did upset the development of the hypothalamus in the DES daughter, then her abnormal hormone balance might upset development of the hypothalamus in her own fetus, so that her daughter (or son?) would grow up with abnormal hormone balance and a predisposition to develop cancer. Therefore, the first experiment should be to find out which of these two mechanisms explains the third generation effect seen in the mouse study. A clear resolution of this problem should be possible with embryo transfer experiments.

Germ cells or Hypothalamus?

If germ cell mutation accounts for third generation cancer, then the cancer risk will follow the embryo made from a mutated egg, regardless of whether or not the embryo develops in the DES daughter mouse that conceived it. Therefore, the critical test is to transfer this embryo to the uterus of a non-DES mouse and see if it still develops DES cancer when it grows up. If so, then the transmission is genetic through the germ cells. A complementary experiment is to transfer a normal embryo into the uterus of a DES daughter mouse. If this embryo later develops DES cancer, then the cancer effect is from transplacental factors, like hormones, that upset development of some part of the fetus, such as the hypothalamus. I have already made these two kinds of embryo transfer (with grant support from the National Cancer Institute) and am currently waiting to see which embryos grow up to have the DES third generation type of cancer. Presumably, the answer will be clearly either a germ cell mechanism or a maternal effect (although the complexities of biological systems can easily upset such an optimistic expectation).

Early Warning

The purpose of finding how the third generation effect is transmitted is to eventually find early signs of an eventual cancer outcome. If something is different about the granddaughter mouse, we could look for this same change in the human DES granddaughter. If it was missing, we could stop worrying. If it was present, we could search for ways to correct it. What is "it". Perhaps an abnormally functioning hypothalamus, if the maternal route is established. If the germ cell route is established, this would not offer any hint as to how the mutated genes were acting. One approach would be to compare the DES granddaughter mouse with a control mouse in many different ways. If the maternal route is the correct explanation for a third generation effect, then I would like to study the hypothalamus for evidence of abnormalities.

Cancer Risk in DES Daughters

A low fat diet may benefit DES daughters directly, as well as protecting DES grand-daughters. My reasoning for this is somewhat indirect. Some physicians are concerned that

DES-related cancer may increase when DES daughters pass menopause. Reproductive tract cancer normally reaches a peak later in life and this same effect was encountered with mice exposed prenatally to DES. In the mouse experiment, endometrial cancer was more common than the cervical and vaginal cancer currently seen in DES daughters. I proposed using the mouse model to screen for ways to prevent this late-occurring increase in uterine cancer, but was unable to raise the necessary funds. Nevertheless, risk factors for endometrial cancer in the general population are well established and could be used to plan a preventive strategy. A major risk factor is obesity. In Chapter Eight I explained how a low fat diet, and diet control generally, can help in avoiding obesity. Therefore, avoiding both high fat intake and obesity in anticipation of pregnancy should benefit both mother and child. Since the link between obesity and uterine cancer is based on studies of the general population, the benefit of avoiding obesity applies to all women and not just to DES daughters.

Relevance of DES Research

Several million people are directly involved in the DES exposure problem. Yet, most people are not in one of the DES exposed generations. Does DES research have any value to people who have never been linked to any kind of DES exposure? I predicted years ago that research on the DES problem would lead to a better understanding of reproductive system cancer in women generally and not just in DES-exposed women. The research I have done on effects of high dietary fat during pregnancy is a direct extension of my research on the DES problem. I believe it is the beginning of a broad new approach to cancer which will benefit everyone eventually.

Women and Cancer

Figures on major causes of death for men and women of various ages were assembled from government sources and published by the American Cancer Society in 1988. Under age 35, the major cause of death for women was accidents, with cancer being second. In the age groups of 35 to 54, and 55 to 74, cancer was the major cause of death. It was not until the age group above 74 that heart disease surpassed cancer. Thus, throughout most years of a woman's life the most lethal disease is cancer. A massive research effort is directed at finding a cure for metastatic cancer, but this goal is proving very difficult to achieve. Meanwhile, cancer prevention provides an alternative. The logical approach to prevention is to first discover the cause, then try to block the process. Of course, how to prevent reproductive system cancer in the next generation is what this book has been all about. The issue I am now raising is how to prevent this type of cancer in women already exposed prenatally to high fat.

Much is already known about the cause of the

major cancers in women. The most common source of cancer in women is the reproductive system. Most risk factors for this type of cancer pertain to the functioning of reproduction and are believed to reflect hormone balance in the body. The major environmental factor for breast, ovarian and endometrial cancer is dietary fat, which probably acts by altering hormone balance. The most likely time for a dietary fat effect is before birth. Therefore, the next step in finding out how to prevent reproductive system cancer in women is to discover how prenatal exposure to fat modifies hormone balance and how this causes cancer later in life. Of course, no research has been done yet on this hypothetical sequence of events. Now that an animal model has been developed, the potential for rapid progress exists.

It may be very difficult to discover exactly what dietary fat does to the fetus and how these changes in the fetus later translate to cancer. Developing effective intervention methods may take a long time. Yet, the converse could be equally true. Working out the mechanism of fat-induced cancer may be well within the scope of current scientific methodology. Once the mechanism is revealed, prevention may prove to be obvious and easy. Considering that cancer is the major cause of death in women throughout most years of their life, and considering that the major source of cancer in women is the reproductive system, shouldn't a massive research effort be launched immediately?

Objections could be raised. Direct proof of a prenatal dietary fat effect is based on a single experiment with mice, which may prove to be faulty in some respect. Epidemiologists have not yet had time to evaluate this new hypothesis and to test it. These are valid objections. The issue is whether they will be used as excuses to do nothing, or whether all pertinent questions will be pursued vigorously. It has taken me five years to raise substantial government funds to do research on the effects of prenatal exposure to dietary fat. Will this be the pace for the future too? Surely the major issue in avoiding premature death for half the people in this nation deserves a more vigorous attack. Is anyone listening?

What About Testing?

Since DES and high dietary fat can program the fetus for cancer later in life, should we now be testing other agents for a similar effect? Such tests are expensive and time-consuming, so the agents would need to be selected carefully. One obvious criterion is the number of babies being exposed. By this criterion ultrasound is of interest, since one to two million fetuses are exposed every year. So far, ultrasound appears to be harmless. Millions of sonicated babies have been born and there is no suggestion of an increase in birth defects. Furthermore, one study looked for an increase in childhood cancer and found no effect. Therefore, it may seem reasonable to assume that ultrasound is also harmless in relation to programming for adult cancer. The issue is whether this assumption justifies waiting 40 years to see for sure that ultrasound has no effect on cancer rate in the adult. That is how long it will take the babies that have already been sonicated to reach the usual age for cancer. Meanwhile, another 40 to 80 million babies will be exposed while we wait for final evidence of safety. I believed such a wait was too big a gamble, so submitted a grant application to the government in 1985 to test for a transplacental carcinogenesis effect of ultrasound in mice. The application was rejected for what I considered to be some very good reasons, including need for collaboration with an electrical engineer. Such collaboration was arranged and we submitted a considerably more sophisticated application in 1987. It was turned down again, this time for some not so very good reasons. I still believe it is not enough to assume ultrasound is safe, we need to prove it is safe. Everything under the sun is tested for birth defects, but almost nothing for fetal programming of adult cancer. The lesson of DES has not yet been learned. Wake up, America.

Appendix

INTRODUCTION TO TABLES

The first table, extending from page 148 to page 183, lists the energy components of a variety of foods. Foods are listed alphabetically in the left column. Note qualifications like fresh, cooked, chopped. The second column lists a quantity, usually corresponding to a serving size or recipe size. If your serving is a different size, be sure to proportionately increase or decrease the amount of fat in the next column labelled FAT, GRAMS. However, the percent fat in the next (fourth) column does not depend on quantity, so is always the same. To use the table, add up the grams of fat in your food, as listed in the third column. To recognize high fat foods, scan down the fourth column, labelled FAT, %. Any food over 30% fat would exceed the recommended level of fat if eaten alone. However, foods with fat content above the 30% level may be satisfactory if eaten with lower fat foods, as explained in Chapters Four through Six. The specific values for protein (PROT), and carbohydrate (CARBO), are expressed in grams and can be copied into tables for analyzing mixtures, recipes and meals. The last column, labelled CAL, shows the total number of calories for the quantity of food listed.

Equivalent measurements for working with recipes are shown below:

1 quart = 2 pints = 4 cups = 32 fluid ounces (fl oz)
1 cup = 8 fluid ounces = 16 tablespoons (tbsp)
1 fluid ounce = 2 tablespoons = 30 milliliters (ml)
1 tablespoon = 3 teaspoons (tsp) = 15 milliliters
1 pound = 16 ounces (oz) = 453.6 grams (gm)
1 ounce = 28.35 grams

Foods with a substantial content of vitamin A in relation to the recommended daily allowance are shown on pages 184 and 187. The percent of recommended daily allowance is shown in the last column with the title %RDA. A similar selection of foods with substantial vitamin C content is found on pages 188 to 193.

These tables of food values are based on a more extensive set of tables prepared for the United States Department of Agriculture. The original tables do not contain a column listing percent fat, but do contain additional listings of nutrients and a greater selection of foods. The percent fat can be calculated from the government publication by multiplying the grams of fat by 9 and dividing this number by the total calories, as explained in Chapter Five. These tables can be ordered as a booklet entitled *NUTRITIVE VALUE OF FOODS*, Home and Garden Bulletin Number 72, for about $4.50. To order, write to:

Superintendent of Documents
U.S. Government Printing Office
Washington, D.C. 20402.

A similar book of tables may be available from local bookstores on special order. It is entitled *HANDBOOK OF THE NUTRITIONAL CONTENTS OF FOODS*, by Bernice K. Watt and Annabel L. Merrill and is published by Dover Publications, Inc., New York. A book currently displayed by many bookstores is *"FOOD VALUES OF PORTIONS COMMONLY USED"* by Pennington and Church. This is a very extensive listing of foods, including some brand name products. It has a section on items served by fast food restaurants. Listings for each food item include calories (KCAL), weight, protein, carbohydrate and fat. Fat content is further defined as polyunsaturated and saturated fatty acids and cholesterol. Other components listed are fiber, vitamins and minerals.

Many commercially packaged foods list the grams of fat, protein and carbohydrate on the package label. These figures should be used in preference to those listed in the following tables, since they are more accurate for that particular product. However, statements like "low fat" or "4% fat " are not useful. If the label does not list grams of fat and total calories, then use the following tables. If the product is a mixture of unknown proportions and cannot be analysed, then look for a comparable product from another company that does list the amounts of each ingredient.

FOOD	MEASURE	FAT GRAMS	FAT %	PROT	CARBO	CAL
Abalone	1 oz	0	0	5	1	28
Almonds, chopped	1 cup	70	76%	24	25	775
Apple juice	1 cup	0	0	0	30	120
Apples, raw	1 apple	1	10%	0	20	80
Apricots, fresh	3 apricots	0	0	1	14	55
Apricots. dried	1 cup	1	2%	7	86	340
Asparagus, cooked	1 cup	0	0	3	5	30
Avocado, raw	1 avocado	37	82%	5	13	370
Bacon, cooked	2 slices	8	82%	4	0	85
Bagels, egg	1 bagel	2	12%	6	28	165

Baking powder	1 tsp	0	0	0	1	5
Banana	1 banana	0	0	1	26	100
Barbecue sauce	1 cup	17	61%	4	20	230
Bass, black sea	4 oz	1	9%	22	0	105
Bass, freshwater	4 oz	3	24%	21	0	118
Beans, canned, green	1 cup	0	0	2	7	30
Beans, dry, common	1 cup	1	4%	14	38	210
Beans, dry, Lima	1 cup	1	3%	16	49	260
Beans, fresh, green	1 cup	0	0	2	7	30
Beans, fresh, Lima	1 cup	0	0	10	32	170
Beans, fresh, yellow	1 cup	0	0	2	6	30
Beans, pork, tomato	1 cup	7	20%	16	48	310

Page 149

FOOD	MEASURE	FAT GRAMS	FAT %	PROT	CARBO	CAL
Bean sprouts, fresh	1 cup	0	0	4	7	35
Beef, rib roast	3 oz	33	81%	17	0	375
Beef, lean, roasted	3 oz	7	39%	25	0	165
Beef, ground, lean	3 oz	10	49%	23	0	185
Beef, round steak, lean	3 oz	13	55%	24	0	220
Beef, sirloin steak	3 oz	27	75%	20	0	330
Beef stew	1 cup	11	44%	16	15	220
Beer	12 fl. oz.	0	0	1	14	150
Beets, canned	1 cup	0	0	2	14	60
Beets, cooked	2 beets	0	0	1	7	30

Beet greens	1 cup	0	0	2	5	25
Biscuits, from mix	1 biscuit	3	28%	2	15	90
Blackeye peas, cooked	1 cup	1	5%	13	30	180
Blackberries, fresh	1 cup	1	10%	2	19	85
Blueberries, fresh	1 cup	1	9%	1	22	90
Bluefish, raw	4 oz	4	28%	23	0	132
Bluefish, baked	3 oz	4	29%	22	0	135
Bologna	1 slice	8	86%	3	0	85
Bonito	4 oz	8	40%	27	0	190
Braunschweiger	1 slice	8	78%	4	1	90
Brazil nuts	1 oz	19	86%	4	3	185
Bread, cracked wheat	1 slice	1	13%	2	13	65

FOOD	MEASURE	FAT GRAMS	FAT %	PROT	CARBO	CAL
Bread, crumbs	1 cup	5	12%	13	73	390
Bread, french	1 slice	1	9%	3	19	100
Bread, raisin	1 slice	1	13%	2	13	65
Bread, rye	1 slice	0	0	2	13	60
Bread, white	1 slice	1	13%	2	13	70
Bread, whole wheat	1 slice	1	12%	3	14	65
Breakfast cereal, cold	1 cup	0	0	2	21	95
Breakfast cereal, hot	1 cup	1	8%	4	23	110
Broccoli, cooked	1 cup	0	0	5	7	40
Brussels sprouts, cooked	1 cup	1	12%	7	10	55

Buckwheat flour	1 cup	1	3%	6	78	340
Buffalofish	4 oz	5	36%	20	0	128
Bullhead	4 oz	2	20%	18	0	95
Butter	1 tbsp	12	100%	0	0	100
Butter, whipped	1 tbsp	8	100%	0	0	65
Buttermilk	1 cup	2	18%	8	12	100
Cabbage, cooked	1 cup	0	0	2	6	30
Cabbage, fresh	1 cup	0	0	1	4	15
Cake, angelfood	1 piece	0	0	3	32	135
Cake, chocolate cupcake	1 cupcake	5	33%	2	21	130
Cake, coffee	1 piece	7	27%	5	38	230
Cake, fruitcake	1 slice	2	31%	1	9	55

FOOD	MEASURE	FAT GRAMS	FAT %	PROT	CARBO	CAL
Cake, pound	1 slice	10	56%	2	16	160
Cake, white, choc. icing	1 piece	8	27%	3	45	250
Candy, caramels	1 oz	3	23%	1	22	115
Candy, chocolate	1 oz	9	53%	2	16	145
Candy, fudge	1 oz	3	23%	1	21	115
Candy, hard	1 oz	0	0	0	28	110
Carp	4 oz	5	36%	20	0	130
Carrots, fresh	1 carrot	0	0	1	7	30
Carrots, cooked	1 cup	0	0	1	11	50
Cashew nuts, roasted	1 cup	64	69%	24	41	785

Catfish	4 oz	3	25%	20	0	117
Cauliflower, cooked	1 cup	0	0	3	5	30
Cauliflower, fresh	1 cup	0	0	3	6	31
Celery, fresh	1 stalk	0	0	0	2	5
Cheese, American, process	1 oz	9	77%	6	0	105
Cheese, blue	1 oz	8	72%	6	1	100
Cheese, camembert	1 wedge	9	72%	8	0	115
Cheese, cheddar	1 oz	9	74%	7	0	115
Cheese, cheddar, shredded	1 cup	37	74%	28	1	455
Cheese, cottage	1 cup	10	40%	28	6	235
Cheese, cottage, 1% fat	1 cup	2	12%	28	6	165
Cheese, cream	1 oz	10	88%	2	1	100

FOOD	MEASURE	FAT GRAMS	FAT %	PROT	CARBO	CAL
Cheese, mozzarella	1 oz	7	69%	6	1	90
Cheese, parmesan, grated	1 tbsp	2	69%	2	0	25
Cheese, parmesan, grated	1 cup	30	59%	42	4	455
Cheese, Swiss, process	1 oz	7	66%	7	1	95
Cherries, sour, canned	1 cup	0	0	2	26	105
Cherries, sweet, fresh	10 cherries	0	0	1	12	45
Chicken, roasted, dark	1 oz	2	36%	8	0	50
Chicken, roasted, white	1 oz	1	20%	9	0	47
Chicken, fried	1 oz	3	40%	9	1	71
Chocolate, baking	1 oz	15	75%	3	8	145

Food	Serving					Calories
Chocolate milk	1 cup	8	35%	8	26	210
Chocolate pudding	1 cup	8	21%	9	59	320
Chocolate syrup topping	2 tbsp	5	34%	2	20	125
Chop suey, beef & pork	1 cup	17	50%	26	13	300
Clams, raw	3 oz	1	15%	11	2	65
Coconut, shredded	1 cup	28	85%	3	8	275
Cod, fresh	4 oz	0	0	20	0	89
Cola beverages	12 fl. oz.	0	0	0	37	145
Collards, cooked	1 cup	1	12%	7	10	65
Cookies, brownies	1 brownie	6	55%	1	10	95
Cookies, chocolate chip	4 cookies	12	51%	2	24	205
Cookies, fig bars	4 cookies	3	13%	2	42	200

FOOD	MEASURE	FAT GRAMS	FAT %	PROT	CARBO	CAL
Cookies, gingersnaps	4 cookies	2	16%	2	22	90
Cookies, oatmeal & raisin	4 cookies	8	31%	3	38	235
Cookies, sandwich	4 cookies	9	40%	2	28	200
Cookies, vanilla wafer	10 cookies	6	30%	2	30	185
Corn, 5 inch ear	1 ear	1	7%	4	27	120
Corn, kernels	1 cup	1	6%	5	31	165
Corn, canned, cream	1 cup	2	7%	5	51	210
Corned beef, canned	3 oz	10	51%	22	0	185
Cornmeal, dry	1 cup	5	10%	11	90	435
Crabmeat, canned	1 cup	3	21%	24	1	135

Crackers, graham	2 crackers	1	17%	1	10	55
Crackers, rye	2 crackers	0	0	2	10	45
Crackers, saltine	4 crackers	1	20%	1	8	50
Crayfish	4 oz	0.5	6%	17	1	82
Cream, half & half	1 cup	28	79%	7	10	315
Cream, sour	1 cup	48	86%	7	10	495
Cream, table	1 cup	46	87%	6	9	470
Cream, whipping	1 cup	74	93%	5	7	700
Cream, whipped topping	1 cup	13	76%	2	7	155
Cream, imitation, whipped	1 cup	19	70%	1	17	240
Cucumbers	6 slices	0	0	0	1	5
Custard, baked	1 cup	15	44%	14	29	305

Page 159

FOOD	MEASURE	FAT GRAMS	FAT %	PROT	CARBO	CAL
Danish pastry	1 oz	7	51%	2	13	120
Dates	10 dates	0	0	2	58	220
Dogfish, spiny	4 oz	10	53%	20	0	177
Donuts, cake, plain	1 donut	5	45%	1	13	100
Donuts, yeast, glazed	1 donut	11	50%	3	22	205
Drum, red	4 oz	0.5	5%	20	0	91
Duck, domestic (with skin)	4 oz	26	80%	15	0	303
Eel	4 oz	21	72%	18	0	264
Eggnog, commercial	1 cup	19	49%	10	34	340
Eggs, raw, large	1 egg	6	66%	6	1	80

Eggs, white only	1 egg white	0	0	3	9	15
Eggs, yolk only	1 egg yolk	6	82%	3	0	65
Endive, curly	1 cup	0	0	1	2	10
Filberts, chopped	1 cup	72	83%	14	19	730
Fish sticks, cooked	1 stick	3	49%	5	2	50
Flounder, fresh	4 oz	1	11%	19	0	90
Frankfurter	1 frank	15	81%	7	1	170
Fruit cocktail, canned	1 cup	0	0	1	50	195
Fruit flavored soft drink	12 fl. oz.	0	0	0	45	170
Gelatin dessert	1 cup	0	0	4	34	140
Gelatin, dry	7 grams	0	0	6	0	25
Gin	1.5 fl. oz.	0	0	0	0	95

FOOD	MEASURE	FAT GRAMS	FAT %	PROT	CARBO	CAL
Ginger ale	12 fl. oz.	0	0	0	29	115
Grapefruit, pink	half	0	0	1	13	50
Grapefruit juice, fresh	1 cup	0	0	1	23	95
Grapejuice, frozen, dilute	1 cup	0	0	1	33	135
Grapes, seedless	10 grapes	0	0	0	9	35
Ground beef, 10% fat	patty (3 oz)	10	49%	23	0	185
Ground beef, 21% fat	patty	17	66%	20	0	235
Grouper	4 oz	0.5	5%	22	0	99
Haddock, raw	4 oz	0	0	21	0	89
Haddock, breaded, fried	3 oz	5	34%	17	5	140

Hake	4 oz	0.5	6%	19	0	84
Halibut	4 oz	1	9%	24	0	114
Ham, boiled, sliced	1 oz	5	69%	5	0	65
Heart, beef, cooked	3 oz	5	29%	27	1	160
Herring, salt water	4 oz	13	59%	20	0	200
Herring, lake	4 oz	2	18%	20	0	109
Honey, strained	1 tbsp	0	0	0	17	65
Ice cream	1 cup	14	46%	5	32	270
Ice cream, rich	1 cup	24	60%	4	32	350
Ice cream, soft	1 cup	23	53%	7	38	375
Jams and preserves	1 tbsp	0	0	0	14	55
Jellies	1 tbsp	0	0	0	13	50

FOOD	MEASURE	FAT GRAMS	FAT %	PROT	CARBO	CAL
Kale, cooked	1 cup	1	16%	5	7	45
Kale, frozen	1 cup	1	17%	4	7	40
Lamb chop	3 oz	32	80%	18	0	360
Lamb chop, lean only	2 oz	6	46%	16	0	120
Lamb, leg roast	3 oz	16	62%	22	0	235
Lamb, shoulder roast	3 oz	23	74%	18	0	285
Lard	1 cup	205	100%	0	0	1850
Lard	1 tbsp	13	100%	0	0	115
Lemon, fresh, juice only	1 cup	0	0	1	20	60
Lemonade (from frozen mix)	1 cup	0	0	0	28	105

Lentils, whole, cooked	1 cup	0	0	16	39	210
Lettuce, iceberg, chopped	1 cup	0	0	0	2	5
Lettuce, romaine, chopped	1 cup	0	0	1	2	10
Lima beans, cooked	1 cup	1	3%	16	49	260
Liver, beef, fried	3 oz	9	43%	22	5	195
Lobster	4 oz	2	19%	19	0	103
Macaroni, hot	1 cup	1	5%	7	39	190
Macaroni and cheese	1 cup	22	46%	17	40	430
Mackerel, raw	4 oz	14	59%	22	0	217
Malted milk	1 cup	10	37%	11	27	235
Margarine, regular	1 tbsp	12	100%	0	0	100
Margarine, regular	1 cup	184	100%	2	0	1630

FOOD	MEASURE	FAT GRAMS	FAT %	PROT	CARBO	CAL
Margarine, whipped	1 tbsp	8	100%	0	0	70
Marshmallows	1 oz	0	0	1	23	90
Mayonnaise	1 tbsp	11	100%	0	0	100
Milk, whole (3.3%)	1 cup	8	49%	8	11	150
Milk, 2% (no additives)	1 cup	5	36%	8	12	120
Milk, 1% (no additives)	1 cup	3	25%	8	12	100
Milk, skim (no additives)	1 cup	0	0	8	12	85
Milk, canned, unsweetened	1 cup	19	50%	17	25	340
Milk, canned, sweetened	1 cup	27	24%	24	166	980
Molasses, light	1 tbsp	0	0	0	13	50

Muffins, bran	1 muffin	4	31%	3	17	105
Muffins, corn	1 muffin	4	29%	3	19	125
Mullet	4 oz	8	45%	22	0	165
Mushrooms, fresh, sliced	1 cup	0	0	2	3	20
Mustard, yellow	1 tsp	-	0	-	-	5
Mustard greens, cooked	1 cup	1	20%	3	6	30
Muskmelon (cantaloup)	half melon	0	0	2	20	80
Noodles, egg, cooked	1 cup	2	9%	7	37	200
Noodles, chow mein, canned	1 cup	11	44%	6	26	220
Ocean perch	4 oz	2	17%	22	0	108
Ocean perch, fried breaded	1 fillet	11	53%	16	6	195
Oil, corn	1 cup	218	100%	0	0	1925

Page 167

FOOD	MEASURE	FAT GRAMS	FAT %	PROT	CARBO	CAL
Oil, corn	1 tbsp	14	100%	0	0	120
Oil, olive	1 cup	216	100%	0	0	1910
Oil, safflower	1 tbsp	14	100%	0	0	120
Oil, soybean	1 cup	218	100%	0	0	1925
Oil, soybean-cottonseed	1 cup	218	100%	0	0	1925
Okra pods, cooked	10 pods	0	0	2	6	30
Olives, green, pickled	4 olives	2	100%	0	0	15
Onions, cooked	1 cup	0	0	3	14	60
Onions, fresh, chopped	1 cup	0	0	3	15	65
Orange juice (frozen)	1 cup	0	0	2	29	120

Oranges, fresh	1 orange	0	0	1	16	65
Oysters, raw	1 cup	4	24%	20	8	160
Pancakes, egg & milk used	1 cake	2	29%	2	9	60
Papayas, fresh, cubed	1 cup	0	0	1	14	55
Parsnips, cooked	1 cup	1	8%	2	23	100
Peaches, fresh	1 peach	0	0	1	10	40
Peaches, canned in syrup	1 cup	0	0	1	51	200
Peanut butter	1 tbsp	8	72%	4	3	95
Peanuts, roasted in oil	1 cup	72	72%	37	27	840
Pears, fresh	1 pear	1	8%	1	25	100
Pears, canned in syrup	1 cup	1	4%	1	50	195
Peas, blackeye, dry	1 cup	1	4%	13	35	190

FOOD	MEASURE	FAT GRAMS	FAT %	PROT	CARBO	CAL
Peas, green, canned	1 cup	1	6%	8	29	150
Peas, green, frozen	1 cup	0	0	8	19	110
Peas, split, dry	1 cup	1	4%	16	42	230
Pecans, chopped	1 cup	84	87%	11	17	810
Peppers, sweet, cooked	1 pod	0	0	1	3	15
Perch, yellow	4 oz	1	9%	22	0	103
Pheasant	4 oz	5	32%	24	0	150
Pickles, dill	1 pickle	0	0	0	1	5
Pickles, gherkin	1 pickle	0	0	0	5	20
Pickles, relish, sweet	1 tbsp	0	0	0	5	20

Pie, apple, 7 servings/pie	1 serving	15	38%	3	51	345
Pie, banana cream	1 serving	12	37%	6	40	285
Pie, blueberry	1 serving	15	40%	3	47	325
Pie, custard	1 serving	14	45%	8	30	285
Pie, lemon meringue	1 serving	12	36%	4	45	305
Pie, mince	1 serving	16	38%	3	56	365
Pie, pecan	1 serving	27	48%	6	61	495
Pie, pumpkin	1 serving	15	48%	5	32	275
Pike, northern	4 oz	1	10%	21	0	100
Pike, walleye	4 oz	1	9%	22	0	105
Pineapple, canned chunks	1 cup	0	0	1	49	190
Pineapple, fresh, diced	1 cup	0	0	1	21	80

FOOD	MEASURE	FAT GRAMS	FAT %	PROT	CARBO	CAL
Pineapple juice, canned	1 cup	0	0	1	34	140
Pizza, cheese, 12 inch	1/8 pizza	4	24%	6	22	145
Plums, fresh	1 plum	0	0	0	8	30
Plums, canned	1 cup	0	0	1	56	215
Pompano	4 oz	11	54%	21	0	188
Popcorn, plain	1 cup	0	0	1	5	25
Popcorn, with oil	1 cup	2	43%	1	5	40
Popsicle, 3 fl. oz.	1 popsicle	0	0	0	18	70
Pork, ham roast	3 oz	19	70%	18	0	245
Pork, loin chop	1 chop	25	75%	19	0	305

Pork, roast	3 oz	24	72%	21	0	310
Potato chips	10 chips	8	62%	1	10	115
Potato salad	1 cup	7	25%	7	41	250
Potatoes, baked	1 potato	0	0	4	33	145
Potatoes, french fried	10 fries	7	44%	2	18	135
Potatoes, hash brown	1 cup	18	46%	3	45	345
Potatoes, mashed, milk	1 cup	2	13%	4	27	135
Pretzels, thin, twisted	10 pretzels	3	11%	6	46	235
Prunes, dry	5 prunes	0	0	1	29	110
Prunes, cooked	1 cup	1	3%	2	67	255
Pudding, chocolate	1 cup	12	26%	8	67	385
Pudding, tapioca cream	1 cup	8	33%	8	28	220

Page 173

FOOD	MEASURE	FAT GRAMS	FAT %	PROT	CARBO	CAL
Pumpkin, canned	1 cup	1	10%	2	19	80
Rabbit, wild	4 oz	5	37%	19	0	122
Radishes, fresh	4 radishes	0	0	0	1	5
Raisins, seedless	1 cup	0	0	4	112	420
Raspberries, red, fresh	1 cup	1	11%	1	17	70
Raspberries, red, frozen	10 oz	1	3%	2	70	280
Red snapper	4 oz	1	9%	22	0	106
Rhubarb, cooked & sugar	1 cup	0	0	1	97	380
Rice, white, cooked	1 cup	0	0	4	50	225
Rum	1.5 oz	0	0	0	0	95

Rolls, hamburger	1 roll	2	16%	3	21	120
Rolls, hard	1 roll	2	11%	5	30	155
Rolls, soft	1 roll	2	22%	2	14	85
Root beer, carbonated	12 fl. oz.	0	0	0	39	150
Salad dressing, blue cheese	1 tbsp	8	90%	1	1	75
Salad dressing, French	1 tbsp	6	82%	0	3	65
Salad dressing, low calorie	1 tbsp	1	53%	0	2	15
Salad dressing, Italian	1 tbsp	9	95%	0	1	85
Salad dressing, mayonnaise	1 tbsp	6	87%	0	2	65
Salad dressing, 1000 Island	1 tbsp	8	90%	0	2	80
Salami, cooked	1 slice	7	76%	5	0	90
Salmon, pink, canned	3 oz	5	40%	17	0	120

FOOD	MEASURE	FAT GRAMS	FAT %	PROT	CARBO	CAL
Salmon, King, fresh	4 oz	18	65%	22	0	251
Sardines, canned in oil	3 oz	9	50%	20	0	175
Sauerkraut, canned	1 cup	0	0	2	9	40
Sausage, country style	2 oz	18	82%	9	0	196
Scallop, raw	2 oz	0	0	9	2	46
Scallops, breaded, fried	6 scallops	8	42%	16	9	175
Shad, baked with butter	3 oz	10	53%	20	0	170
Shake, thick, vanilla	11 oz	9	23%	12	56	313
Sheepshead, Atlantic	4 oz	3	23%	23	0	128
Sherbet, 2% fat	1 cup	4	13%	2	59	270

Shortening, vegetable	1 cup	200	100%	0	0	1770
Shortening, vegetable	1 tbsp	13	100%	0	0	110
Smelt	4 oz	2	18%	21	0	111
Shrimp, canned	3 oz	1	9%	21	1	100
Shrimp, raw	4 oz	1	9%	21	2	103
Shrimp, French fried	3 oz	9	44%	17	9	190
Snap beans, green	1 cup	0	0	2	7	30
Soups, canned, condensed:						
Soup, bean & pork, water	1 cup	6	31%	8	22	170
Soup, beef noodle, water	1 cup	3	38%	4	7	65
Soup, chicken with milk	1 cup	10	51%	7	15	180
Soup, chicken with water	1 cup	6	55%	3	8	95

FOOD	MEASURE	FAT GRAMS	FAT %	PROT	CARBO	CAL
Soup, clam chowder, water	1 cup	3	33%	2	12	80
Soup, split pea, water	1 cup	3	18%	9	21	145
Soup, tomato with milk	1 cup	7	34%	7	23	175
Soup, tomato with water	1 cup	3	27%	2	16	90
Soup, vegetable beef	1 cup	2	23%	5	10	80
Soup, vegetarian	1 cup	2	23%	2	13	80
Soups, dehydrated:						
Soup, chicken noodle	1 cup	1	18%	2	8	55
Soup, onion	1 cup	1	24%	1	6	35
Soup, tomato vegetable	1 cup	1	15%	1	12	65

Food	Serving					Calories
Spaghetti, cooked, tender	1 cup	1	6%	5	32	155
Spaghetti, sauce, cheese	1 cup	9	31%	9	37	260
Spaghetti, canned	1 cup	2	9%	6	39	190
Spaghetti, sauce, meat	1 cup	12	32%	19	39	330
Spinach, canned	1 cup	1	15%	6	7	50
Spinach, cooked	1 cup	1	17%	5	6	40
Spinach, fresh	1 cup	0	0	2	2	15
Squash, summer, cooked	1 cup	0	0	2	7	30
Squash, winter, cooked	1 cup	1	6%	4	32	130
Strawberries, fresh	1 cup	1	14%	1	13	55
Strawberries, frozen	10 oz	1	3%	1	79	310
Sugar, brown, packed	1 cup	0	0	0	212	820

FOOD	MEASURE	FAT GRAMS	FAT %	PROT	CARBO	CAL
Sugar, white, granulated	1 cup	0	0	0	199	770
Sugar, white, granulated	1 tbsp	0	0	0	12	45
Sugar, powdered, sifted	1 cup	0	0	0	100	385
Sunflower seeds, dry	1 cup	69	71%	35	29	810
Sweetpotato, baked	1 potato	1	5%	2	37	160
Swordfish	4 oz	4	29%	22	0	134
Tangerine, fresh	1 tangerine	0	0	1	10	40
Tartar sauce	1 tbsp	8	95%	0	1	75
Toaster pastries	1 pastry	6	26%	3	36	200
Tomato catsup	1 tbsp	0	0	0	4	15

Tomato juice	1 cup	0	0	2	10	45
Tomatoes, canned	1 cup	0	0	2	10	50
Tomatoes, fresh	1 tomato	0	0	1	6	25
Tomcod, Atlantic, raw	4 oz	0.5	6%	19	0	87
Trout, lake	4 oz	23	76%	16	0	273
Trout, rainbow	4 oz	13	55%	24	0	221
Tuna, fresh	4 oz	5	28%	29	0	165
Tuna, canned in oil	3 oz	7	40%	24	0	170
Tuna, canned in water	3 oz	1	9%	22	0	100
Turkey, roasted, dark	3 oz	7	38%	26	0	175
Turkey, roasted, white	3 oz	3	19%	28	0	150
Turnips, cooked	1 cup	0	0	1	8	35

FOOD	MEASURE	FAT GRAMS	FAT %	PROT	CARBO	CAL
Turnip greens	1 cup	0	0	3	5	30
Veal cutlet, cooked	3 oz	9	47%	23	0	185
Veal rib roast	3 oz	14	58%	23	0	230
Venison, lean meat	4 oz	5	32%	24	0	143
Vinegar, cider	1 tbsp	0	0	0	1	3
Waffles	1 waffle	8	35%	7	27	205
Walnuts, black, chopped	1 cup	74	79%	26	19	785
Walnuts, English (Persian)	1 cup	77	82%	18	19	780
Watermelon, fresh	1 wedge	1	7%	2	27	110
Weakfish	4 oz	6	42%	19	0	137

Wheat flour, all-purpose	1 cup	1	2%	12	88	420
Wheat flour, pastry	1 cup	1	3%	7	76	350
Wheat flour, whole-wheat	1 cup	2	4%	16	85	400
Whisky, 80-proof	1 1/2 oz	0	0	0	0	95
Whitefish, lake	4 oz	9	49%	21	0	176
Whiting	4 oz	3	24%	21	0	119
Wine, dessert	3 1/2 oz	0	0	0	8	140
Wine, table	3 1/2 oz	0	0	0	4	85
Yeast, baker's	7 gm	0	0	3	3	20
Yellowtail	4 oz	6	36%	24	0	156
Yogurt, low fat, fruit	8 oz	3	11%	10	42	230
Yogurt, low fat, plain	8 oz	4	24%	12	16	145
Yogurt, whole milk	8 oz	7	45%	8	11	140

FOODS FOR VITAMIN A	MEASURE	UNITS	%RDA (5000 UNITS)
Apricots, raw	3 apricots	2890	58
Apricots, dried	3 apricots	1400	28
Asparagus	1 cup	1310	26
Avocado, raw	1 avocado	630	13
Beans, Lima	1 cup	400	8
Beans, green	1 cup	680	14
Beet greens, cooked	1 cup	7400	148
Broccoli	1 cup	3880	78
Brussel sprouts	1 cup	810	16
Butter	1 tbsp	430	9

Cantaloup (orange)	1 pound	7710	154
Carrots, raw	1 carrot	7930	159
Cereal	1 oz.	see label	0 to 100%
Chard, Swiss, raw	1 oz.	1695	34
Collards, cooked	1 cup	14820	296
Corn, kernels	1 cup	580	12
Endive, raw	1 cup	1650	33
Ice cream	1 cup	540	11
Kale, cooked	1 cup	9130	183
Lettuce, romaine	1 cup	1050	21
Liver, beef	3 oz.	45390	908
Margarine	1 tbsp	470	9

Page 185

Good Sources of Vitamin A

FOODS FOR VITAMIN A	MEASURE	UNITS	%RDA (5000 UNITS)
Milk	1 cup	see label	about 10%
Mustard greens, cooked	1 cup	8120	162
Orange juice	1 cup	500	10
Papayas, raw	1 cup	2450	49
Peaches, raw, yellow flesh	1 peach	1330	27
Peaches, canned	1 cup	1100	22
Peas, green, canned	1 cup	1170	23
Prunes, dried	5 prunes	690	14
Pumpkin, canned	1 cup	15680	314
Spaghetti sauce	4 oz.	see label	about 10

Spinach, raw	1 cup	4460	89
Spinach, cooked	1 cup	14580	292
Squash, summer, cooked	1 cup	820	16
Squash, baked, winter	1 cup	8610	172
Sweetpotatoes, baked	1 potato	9230	185
Tomatoes, raw	1 tomato	1110	22
Tomato juice	1 cup	1940	39
Tomato soup with milk	1 cup	1200	24
Turnip greens, cooked	1 cup	8270	165
Vegetables, mixed, frozen	1 cup	9010	180
Vegetarian soup with water	1 cup	2940	59

FOODS FOR VITAMIN C	MEASURE	MILLIGRAMS	%RDA (60 mg.)
Apples, raw	1 apple	6	10
Apricots, raw	3 apricots	11	18
Asparagus, cooked	4 spears	16	27
Avocados	1 avocado	30	50
Banana	1 banana	12	20
Beans, Lima, cooked	1 cup	29	48
Beans, green, cooked	1 cup	15	25
Beans, yellow, cooked	1 cup	16	27
Bean sprouts, raw	1 cup	20	33
Beets, cooked	2 beets	6	10

Beet greens, cooked	1 cup	22	37
Blackberries, raw	1 cup	30	50
Blackeye peas, cooked	1 cup	28	47
Blueberries, raw	1 cup	20	33
Broccoli, cooked	1 stalk	162	270
Brussels sprouts, cooked	1 cup	135	225
Cabbage, raw	1 cup	33	55
Cabbage, cooked	1 cup	48	80
Carrots, raw	1 carrot	6	10
Cantaloup, orange-fleshed	1 pound	74	123
Cauliflower, raw, chopped	1 cup	90	150
Cauliflower, cooked	1 cup	69	115

FOODS FOR VITAMIN C	MEASURE	MILLIGRAMS	%RDA (60 mg.)
Cereal	1 oz.	see label	0-100
Cherries, sweet, raw	10 cherries	7	12
Collards, cooked	1 cup	144	240
Corn, kernels, cooked	1 cup	8	13
Corn, canned, creamed	1 cup	13	22
Grapefruit, raw	1/2 grapefruit	44	73
Grapefruit juice	1 cup	93	155
Kale, cooked	1 cup	102	170
Lemon, raw	1 lemon	39	65
Lettuce, romaine, raw	1 cup	10	17

Liver, beef, fried	3 oz.	23	38
Mustard greens, cooked	1 cup	67	112
Okra pods, cooked	10 pods	21	35
Onions, raw	1 cup	15	25
Onions, cooked	1 cup	17	28
Oranges	1 orange	66	110
Orange juice	1 cup	124	207
Papayas, raw	1 cup	78	130
Parsnips, cooked	1 cup	16	27
Peaches, raw	1 peach	7	12
Pears, raw	1 pear	7	12
Peas, green, canned	1 cup	14	23

FOODS FOR VITAMIN C	MEASURE	MILLIGRAMS	%RDA (60 mg.)
Pineapple, raw	1 cup	26	43
Pineapple, canned	1 slice	7	12
Potatoes, baked	1 potato	31	52
Raspberries, raw	1 cup	31	52
Rhubarb, cooked	1 cup	16	27
Sauerkraut, canned	1 cup	33	55
Spinach, raw	1 cup	28	47
Spinach, cooked	1 cup	50	83
Squash, cooked	1 cup	21	35
Strawberries, raw	1 cup	88	147

Sweetpotatoes, baked	1 potato	25	42
Tangerine, raw	1 tangerine	27	45
Tomatoes, raw	1 tomato	28	47
Tomato juice	1 cup	39	65
Tomato soup	1 cup	15	25
Turnips, cooked	1 cup	34	57
Turnip greens	1 cup	68	113
Vegetables, mixed, frozen	1 cup	15	25